EATING YOUR MEDITATION

Cover: In 1990, Mark Harrington took a picture of the neon sign at the entrance to the Santa Fe Super Chief Railcar Diner when it was still in business and parked in Santa Fe on Guadalupe street. Soon after Mr. Harrington took the photo, the diner closed and the railcar was retired to the Santa Fe train yard. In 2003, Mr. Harrington used this photo to make the mandala featured on the cover.

EATING YOUR MEDITATION

A Guide to Metamorphic Nutrition

Steven Roberts

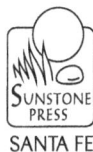

SUNSTONE
PRESS

SANTA FE

Grateful acknowledgement is made to Mark Harrington
for permission to use his mandala on the cover.
The artist's mandala was further inspired by M.C. Escher—Heirs c/o Cordon
Art-Baarn, The Netherlands © Kaleidocycles.

Thanks to Greg Whiteley for permission to use
the trademarked term Solar Nutrition.

Please contact the author at P.O. Box 22702, Santa Fe, New Mexico 87502

Sunstone books may be purchased for educational, business, or sales promotional use. For
information please write: Special Markets Department, Sunstone Press,
P.O. Box 2321, Santa Fe, New Mexico 87504-2321.

Library of Congress Cataloging-in-Publication Data

Roberts, Steven, 1952 July 30-
    Eating your meditation : a guide to metamorphic nutrition / [Steven
Roberts].
       p. cm.
    Includes bibliographical references and index.
    ISBN 0-86534-415-9 (pbk.)
    1. Nutrition—Miscellanea. 2. Self-care, Health. 3. Light—Therapeutic use. I. Title.
RA784 .R585 2003
613.2—dc22
                        2003017492

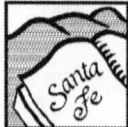

Published in

SUNSTONE PRESS
POST OFFICE BOX 2321
SANTA FE, NM 87504-2321 / USA
(505) 988-4418 / ORDERS ONLY (800) 243-5644
FAX (505) 988-1025
WWW.SUNSTONEPRESS.COM

To my wife Linda, who introduced me to eating Solar. This book is as much yours as it is mine. Thank you for all your help and the last sixteen years of Solar meals.

I also dedicate this work to Adano. I pray I have faithfully shared your lessons with those who have yet to meet you.

Because I was asked . . .

CONTENTS

PREFACE -- 9

INTRODUCTION TO EATING SOLAR ---------------------------------- 13

FIVE SOLAR RULES --- 25

    1. A little bit of ANYTHING is medicine, too much is TOXIC (abuse).27

    2. There is a TIME, a PLACE, and a SEASON for EVERYTHING. ------ 35

    3. Live to EAT to get SICK. --- 41

    4. Live to EAT NOT to GET SICK. ------------------------------------- 49

    5. LIVE TO EAT in order to LIVE *NOT* TO EAT (MEMORY PATTERN). 65

HOW TO EAT YOUR MEDITATION -------------------------------- 75

    ZONE ONE: Dawn to 12 noon ------------------------------------- 81

    ZONE TWO: 12 noon to 6 p.m. ----------------------------------- 83

    ZONE THREE: 6 p.m. to 9 p.m. ----------------------------------- 85

    CROSSOVER: 11:30 a.m. to 12 noon and 5:30 p.m. to 6 p.m. ------- 87

    A FEW BASICS -- 89

    FOOD PREPARATION -- 91

    BLOOD TYPE -- 101

    BUYER BE AWARE -- 105

MAHASANA -- 113

ADANO and SOLAR NUTRITION --------------------------------- 119

LIST OF REFERENCES -- 127

PREFACE

An extraordinary person named Adano C. Ley taught us how to eat for maximum assimilation, cellular regeneration, and environmental synchronicity. He gave us the rules for living. We learned that *when* we eat is as important as what we eat.

When we eat food, the KEY ingredient we take in is LIGHT. When we eat *on time*, our bodies absorb the maximum amount of LIGHT from the food. Therefore, we select food in accord with how much LIGHT it receives. The sun dictates when we eat, so we call it eating *Solar* or *Eating Your Meditation*, because we take every bite with awareness. Some meditation techniques pay special attention to the breath with increased awareness. We pay special attention to how much LIGHT the food contains by being aware of its growth cycle.

For example, nuts and fruits that grow high in the trees receive the maximum amount of sunlight early in the day. So we eat nuts and fruits such as prunes, almonds, peaches, and apples in the morning. At 12 noon, vegetables that grow four inches above the ground to four feet high get the maximum amount of sunlight. This is the time to eat vegetables such as squash, lettuce, peppers, eggplant, tomatoes, broccoli, and cauliflower. We also eat two-leggeds such as chicken and turkey, and four-leggeds such as beef and buffalo in the afternoon. Between 6 p.m. and 12 midnight, we eat foods that grow in the bounce light range such as fish, eggs, beets, carrots, and potatoes. During each time frame the body produces the necessary digestive enzymes to fully assimilate food eaten on time, and our food is rapidly and thoroughly absorbed.

Your body is the car you drive through life. Eating food in accord with its light cycle sets the timing for your body, like setting the timing in an automobile. If you eat out of time, you will be out of time mechanically and your health will suffer. Thus, your health is timing.

Another name for timing is *synchronicity*. The environment was put here before us and we are thrown into It to learn how to synchronize with It. Another name for the environment is God. The ancients stated this principle as, "Not my will, but Thy Will be done."

Moreover, the simple act of eating on time can change every CELL in your physical body into pure LIGHT. Because LIGHT does not decompose, immortality of the human mechanism is possible. You can become something completely NEW right NOW.

When we graduate from the school of NOW, we receive our **SMS** degree. The first **S** stands for sane or saint. The **M** stands for millionaire or money manager, because we pay our bills ahead of time, with plenty to spare and plenty to share, no matter what the number. The last **S** in our **SMS** degree stands for student/scientist, because we are always learning.

INTRODUCTION TO EATING SOLAR

From 1998-2001, I lived in Phoenix, Arizona. The Gila River Indian Reservation is 30 miles south of Phoenix off State Highway 347. For over two thousand years, the indigenous Pima people lived near the Gila River and farmed the land in southern Arizona. In the early years of the 20th century, white settlers in Phoenix diverted the upper waters of the Gila River for their own use. The Pima people's irrigation canals dried up and the land died. The Pima people lost their link to the land and needed government help to survive.

Times were hard for these people until 1984, when the Arizona state legislature approved gambling casinos on reservation land. With a monopoly on gambling in this rich state, the indigenous Pima people once again prospered. Having lost their link to the land long ago, they eagerly embraced the American mainstream culture.

The Pima build their homes with the same materials as typical houses found in any Phoenix neighborhood. They dress the same as most Americans, eat at McDonald's, and shop at Wal-Mart. For all practical purposes, they have assimilated into the American way of life and eat the modern American diet.

Yet the Pima people on the reservation face a serious health crisis. Over half of them are severely obese. Most suffer from diseases linked to obesity such as hypertension, birth defects, muscle strains, back problems, joint disorders, sleep apnea, high blood pressure, several forms of cancer, and the largest killer; diabetes. Sixty percent of Pima adults are diabetic, with more children and adults developing diabetes daily. The top two killers of diabetics are stroke and heart disease.

Gambling profits built the Pima people a state-of-the-art hospital to deal with the mounting health problems. The kidney dialysis clinic operates fourteen hours a day, six days a week, treating 18 patients at once. Still, this is not enough to keep up with demand in this small community. The Pima Native Americans in southern Arizona hold the unwelcome distinction of being the fattest people in the fattest country on Earth.

About one thousand years ago, some Pima people split from the main tribe and left southern Arizona. They settled 500 miles to the south in the Sierra Madre mountains of northern Mexico. The Mexican Pima farm by the river and live off the land with no electricity, no piped water, and few modern conveniences. They live in tune with Nature, eating a traditional diet of fruit, vegetables, and corn tortillas. They are fit and healthy. Researchers note that diabetes and obesity are virtually unknown there. The Sierra Madre Pima are, on average, 60 pounds lighter than their Arizona cousins. (Anthony Thomas, *Frontline* 1708 "FAT," air date on PBS: November 3, 1998)

By observing the remarkable physical difference between the two branches of the Pima Nation we can see how modern living affects our health. Experts say obesity is surpassing malnutrition as the primary dietary concern worldwide. The medical establishment considers two-thirds of the people in the United States overweight or obese. Furthermore, the number of overweight people in America *doubles* every seven years, and the number of overweight people becoming seriously obese continues to rise. Currently, forty-five million Americans are *seriously* obese. One-quarter of American children are obese, more than twice the number two decades ago. With each passing day, more children suffer from type 2 diabetes, a disease that once struck only middle age adults. Obesity is the second leading cause of death in the United States. Smoking is number one. "The CDC estimates that about 280,000 Americans die every year as a direct result of being overweight." (Schlosser, p.241)

The United States food industry is the third largest global industry—ahead of computers, aerospace, and electronics. Food is an industrial product marketed through aggressive advertising campaigns. Ninety-five percent of the food industry's commercials advertise foods dense in processed salt, refined sugar, and saturated fat. Clever television commercials aimed at adults and innocent children promote candy, soft drinks, sugar-coated cereals, and fast foods such as hamburgers and pizza.

The typical American fast food diet nutritionally starves the body. You eat and eat and eat and still feel hungry. As the years go by, you gain more weight. If you try to starve the body on a calorie reduction program to lose weight, your body will fight to survive by maintaining stores of fat. When you return to your normal eating habits, the body thinks it is still starving because it lacks nourishment and it will store even more fat. Whether you diet or eat normally your body keeps storing fat. As the saying goes, "You can't win for losing."

An endless stream of new diets, weight reduction pills, nutritional supplements, and exercise gadgets tempt desperate overweight people. Granted, dieting causes loss of fat. Yet dieting also causes loss of bone, muscle, water, and electrolytes. Dieting develops fat-depositing enzymes that increase the risk for heart disease. When faced with starvation, the mind and body will fight to maintain fat. Consequently, the dieter needs superhuman willpower to fight the body's cries for nourishment.

Under the pressure from a fictional society portrayed in print and on television, it is no wonder the dieter's willpower falters. As soon as the diet ends, they return to their previous behavior pattern and gain back all the weight they lost. Anyone with experience dieting will tell you, "Diets don't work!" Countless studies show that 95 percent of dieters regain all the weight they lost within two years. Diets don't work because a diet does not permanently change behavior. At best, a diet is a temporary fix. Most dieters look forward to the day they can go off their diet and return to their normal eating habits, the behavior that got them in trouble in the first place!

Eating Solar presents a new approach to weight control by breaking our addiction to food. Solar eating involves discipline, not willpower. Willpower crumbles under the pressure from your starving CELLS and the food industry's relentless programming to eat 'comfort' foods. Discipline is much easier, because your body supports it. Your body wants to eat the right foods at the right time, because it wants nourishment. Just the same, your body will object when you eat the wrong foods at the wrong time. Thus, your CELLS teach you to discipline yourself. Discipline means selecting the right foods at the right time of day.

The word *discipline* comes from the word *disciple*. A disciple is a devoted student or follower of certain rules. Rules are nothing more than tools, or guidelines for living. For example, to drive a car safely we must learn the rules of the road. Once we learn the rules of the road, we are free to enjoy the journey. Rules are the road map we follow and the road itself.

This book gives you five Solar rules for eating on time as taught by Adano. With the correct knowledge about how to eat what foods when, you learn how to select the right foods at the right time of day. When you eat foods on time your body metabolizes food easily, you get maximum nutrition from the food, and your behavior permanently changes. You discipline yourself to follow the rules of the road for optimum health and your body supports it. Because you are no longer dieting and starving your CELLS, you calm down. You become less hyper and more compassionate. The food and the sunlight in the food, automatically synchronize your body to Nature's metamorphic process. You discover that discipline leads to freedom.

In the wild, there is no obesity crisis. Animals are in balance with Nature. Modern society insulates us from Nature and tries to impose its will upon Nature. When you eat Solar, you balance your CELLS with Nature. Eating Solar works with your body's natural rhythm rather than fighting against it. Nature becomes your friend, not your enemy. You begin to connect with Nature, and It becomes your guide and teacher.

If you are overweight and eat Solar, weight loss happens as a natural *side-effect*. You can eat in the right time frame, or on time, and still lose weight, because the body metabolizes the food more efficiently. Therefore, calories are meaningless to the Solar eater. Solar eaters do not count calories. Solar eaters select foods in accord with the amount of LIGHT in the food, not calorie count.

When you eat Solar, your weight automatically stabilizes to your body's *functional weight*. Your functional weight is the diameter of your wrist multiplied by your height in inches. If you need to gain weight to achieve your functional weight, you will. If you need to lose weight to achieve your functional weight, you will. The Solar process is automatic self-cleaning and self-regulating. Your body achieves balance because you are in accord with Nature.

When it comes to eating, TIME is the important factor. What you eat is also important, but timing overrides what you eat. Eating on time offers the body maximum nutrition and assimilation from the food. Eating Solar works with the body's natural digestive cycles which allow the body to selectively extract the highest amount of nourishment from the food and discard the rest. Thus your body receives the vitamins and minerals it needs *when* it needs them. Consequently, you no longer starve.

Sadly, most people are unaware of the role timing plays in reference to their health. So they eat out of time. In America we suffer from potluck eating, not malnutrition. When we eat at the wrong time, our bodies struggle to absorb food. Eating Solar, on the other hand, plugs you into Nature's flow like plugging an electric cord into a light socket. When you are in the flow, you are in sync with the environment, your CELLS receive the nourishment they need, and subtle changes start to manifest.

Our body is a collection of constantly changing CELLS. The average person depletes their cell bank at the rate of five million cells a second. In other words, five million cells die and five million cells are reborn every second. In addition, our body replaces every cell in seven years. So every seven years we change into a new person. But what do we change into?

The environment gives us the caterpillar and the butterfly as models for the cellular change happening within us. The caterpillar symbolizes the decomposing state of the mechanism. The butterfly symbolizes the non-decomposing state of the mechanism.

Most of us are like the caterpillar. We eat what we want, when we want. The caterpillar eats everything put in front of it and is everyone's enemy. It destroys the plants and trees it feeds on. If the caterpillar refuses to stop devouring plants after forty days, it will die a final death into its own extinction. Most of us eat everything put in front of us, just like the caterpillar, and die a similar death, ignorant of our higher nature. If you step on a caterpillar, the body rots. Similarly, when we die, our body rots.

Yet locked in the caterpillar's DNA is the butterfly. At some point, the wise caterpillar stops eating and decides to change. It spins a cocoon and retires to the darkness where it fasts and waits. Nature begins to transform its body. After 72 hours, a beautiful butterfly emerges from its cocoon and flies away. The butterfly's food waits in the hearts of flowers. It flits from flower to flower enjoying the sublime nectar and delicate tastes of each bloom. The butterfly no longer needs to steal to eat.

Furthermore, if you kill a butterfly, the body does not rot. Collectors admire them, seek after them, and even stick pins into them and hang them on the wall. Still, the butterfly's body does not rot, it is just as beautiful as when it was alive. The butterfly's body is a non-decomposing body type mechanism, an incorruptible body. It does not die, decompose, and return to the earth. The caterpillar's CELLS resurrect into an immortal life. Similarly, we can literally resurrect our CELLS to butterflyhood, or incorruptibility, because the non-decomposing Diamond Body Program is in the DNA of our CELLS.

DNA works in our human body like a hard drive works in a computer. Our DNA contains many different programs or information clusters, including the Diamond Body Program. Messenger RNAs called *ribosomes* read and transcribe the information from the DNA's active programs and translate the program's instructions into what geneticists call "structural proteins." Proteins make up most of what we are. Proteins are the ultimate stuff of life, the biological mud used to build and maintain our CELLS. The active programs on our DNA's hard drive tell the carpenter what to build. And every seven years our divine carpenter builds us a new house, called a BODY, to live in.

The genetic material of all organisms, the DNA, was regarded as a blueprint for the body. Today, however, geneticists understand that DNA is not stagnant with pre-designed functions like a blueprint picture. Instead, geneticists discovered that DNA "within complex organisms interact with other genes and are influenced by their environment." (Hart, p.255) Eating Solar gives our CELLS the right nourishment at the right time, thus altering our DNA's living environment. By changing the DNA's environment, we can unlock the Diamond Body Program stored on our hard drive to awaken the superman, or superwoman within.

Ninety-seven percent of our DNA is a mystery to scientists, so they label it "junk" DNA. It is far from junk. Nature wastes nothing and creates nothing without a purpose. Everything has a reason for being. Our undiscovered DNA is the place on our hard drive where the Diamond Body Program lives. Hence, our junk DNA holds the KEY to humanity's next dramatic evolutionary leap.

At our current stage of development our earthy crystalline body is mostly carbon and silicone, a *carbon-based* body. Our carbon-based body is similar to charcoal, which does not let much light through. When charcoal is subjected to heat and pressure through time, it purifies into a diamond. Diamond lets a lot of light through and is the hardest stone on Earth, indivisible and uncuttable by anything but another diamond. The ancients called the diamond body *vajra yana*. Vajra (pronounced "Benza") means indestructible. Yana means vehicle, or mechanism. The diamond body mechanism is a biologically resurrected carbon body, an indestructible time-space vehicle. The myth of the Savior's death and resurrection in most of the world's religions alludes to this scientific fact living in our CELLS.

When our DNA unlocks the Diamond Body Program it is like the Fourth of July inside the body. Our CELLS transform into the atomic structure of the universe. We recognize our oneness with It. The Diamond Body Program in our DNA *automatically* transforms our CELLS from a carbon-based body type to a diamond-based body type as the caterpillar *automatically* transforms its CELLS into the butterfly. Just like the caterpillar, we are living models of a natural process.

The great Indian mystic and philosopher Sri Aurobindo (1872-1950) said, "Man is a transitional being; he is not final. The next step from man to superman is the next approaching achievement in the earth's evolution. It is inevitable because it is at once the intention of the inner Spirit and the logic of Nature's process." (qtd. in Satprem, *On The Way to Supermanhood*, Institute for Evolutionary Research, New York, 1985)

When your carbon-based body resurrects into the immortal diamond body, you wake up from your robotic conditioned slumber and become conscious of consciousness. You return from a solid state to a magnetic state within your mechanism. Resurrection is a cosmic reality and a science of living, not a religious idea.

Through Nature's evolutionary process of time based reincarnation, we are ever-so-slowly evolving into the incorruptible diamond body. Buried deep within our DNA, carried from one generation to the next, is the seed (the program) for the diamond body. Eating Solar automatically unlocks the Diamond Body Program within our DNA, thus accelerating the carbon body's natural march of evolution through time. By eating Solar, we help our CELLS transform from a decomposing mechanism to a non-decomposing mechanism, right NOW, without waiting for another birth.

Note Well:

What follows are Adano's five Solar Rules and the general principles he used to teach Solar eating. Linda and I have worked with it since 1987. During that time, we have made a few discoveries of our own and included them where appropriate.

FIVE SOLAR RULES

"Don't blame me! I didn't make the rules, I'm stuck with 'em!"

—Adano C. Ley

1. A little bit of ANYTHING is medicine, too much is TOXIC (abuse). —K'ung Fu-Tse, (551-479 BCE) was known as Confucius, the Latinized name for 'Kong the Master.' Adano called him "Corny-fucius."

An Oriental proverb says, "Observe the old, discover the new." When we acknowledge what the ancients observed and apply it NOW, we can discover a new way to live. The ancients saw our bodies as part of the environment. They recognized the sun as the greatest source of health for all life on Earth. The ancients regarded the sun as the giver of light and life, the preserver, and even the Savior of the world. In this regard, the ancients knew that the sun is the KEY to our health and longevity.

The sun has a diameter of 864,000 miles and contains 99 percent of the matter in the solar system. (Gallant, p.37, *Our Universe*, National Geographic Society, 1986) Each day the magnificent sun rises to "save the world" from the darkness of night. If the Earth were cutoff from the sun's rays for a month, all living things would perish and the Earth would revert to a frozen waste. Organisms could not live long without the life-giving rays of the sun. Under the influence of the sun's rays the barren Earth gives forth lush vegetation, trees sprout new leaves, and the oceans produce plankton to feed all within its depths. The sun causes life to flourish.

The sun rotates faster at the equator than at the poles creating incredible electromagnetic waves in the form of solar Life Energy.

Solar energy is the basic source of energy found in fossil fuels, the combustion of wood, even hydroelectric power. Ultraviolet light from the sun reinforces your body's resistance to infections, improves the oxygen carrying capacity of the blood, increases tolerance to stress, decreases blood pressure, reduces your resting heart rate while boosting cardiac output, lowers blood cholesterol, lowers blood sugar, and heightens energy. (Kime, p.46)

Yet, with all the scientifically proven benefits of sunlight, the medical establishment urges us to protect ourselves from the sun with sunglasses and sunscreens. To block the sun's healing rays is counter-productive for health. Avoiding the sun contributes to a weaker immune system.

We must use caution and respect the sun's power to gain the maximum benefit from its healing rays. The sun feeds us mentally, chemically, and spiritually. It nourishes everything. All food depends on the sun's rays to maintain it. When we eat food, we ingest vitamins and minerals as *indirect* sunlight. Eating food in accord with the food's growth cycle, or light cycle (eating Solar) gets the maximum amount of light from food. Whether we know it or not, LIGHT is what we seek from food.

The Solar lifestyle begins with Kung Fu-Tse's statement, "A little bit of anything is medicine, too much is toxic." "Too much" the doctors call *hyper.* "Too little" the doctors call *hypo.* We start to practice the Solar lifestyle "a little bit", which is balance. Later on, we phase into stricter use of the techniques. Eating Solar is a lifelong learning process, not a diet or a quick fix.

The Solar lifestyle starts with sunbathing. You can eat all the finest foods, yet without exposing your CELLS directly to sunlight you risk sickness. When sunlight hits the skin, vitamin D is produced. Vitamin D is not a vitamin as first thought by researchers, but a beneficial hormone that helps to build the body's immunity. Our bodies need Vitamin D to use and assimilate calcium. In addition, when sunlight is *indirectly* exposed to our eyes, it stimulates the pineal gland to secrete melatonin, which has a positive effect on the brain, the adrenals, and the reproductive organs. (Remember: Never look directly at the sun.)

The ancients knew that we are children of the sun and we should expose our skin to its healing rays. Always expose yourself to the sun a little bit, at the right time of day. Too much exposure at the wrong time of day is toxic. The best times to sunbathe are before 10 a.m. and after 4 p.m. The sun's ultraviolet rays pass through large amounts of atmosphere at these times of day and are filtered for safe skin exposure. Limit your exposure. If your skin burns, it is too much. Use hats and light clothing for protection when needed. If you expose your skin to the right amount of sun, your health will benefit in many ways.

Next, the Solar lifestylist learns how to absorb indirect sunlight through food by eating on time. What to eat when remains a mystery to most people because we are disconnected from the environment.

Most people do not know how to eat for health. Eating Solar is the corrective pattern.

A carbon-based body is the vehicle we have to work with. The carbon body is vulnerable to five causes of sickness and disease. They are 1)broken bones, 2)toxic ingestion, 3)genetic disorder, 4)bacterial/viral invasion, and 5)trauma—physical or emotional. The western world offers three kinds of medicine: 1)symptomatic, 2)homeopathic, and 3)placebo.

Symptomatic medicine (also called allopathic medicine) works against the symptoms and uses drugs to overpower them. Most prescribed drugs fight against and cover up symptoms. Therefore, symptomatic medicine is like using a policeman to catch a thief.

Homeopathic medicine uses symptoms to work with the cure; the principle of like curing like. In homeopathy, a remedy gives the body a needed frequency that stimulates and rebalances the mechanism. If the remedy's frequency matches the patient's illness state, a resonant transfer of energy allows the patient's bio-energetic system to assimilate the needed energy, throw off the toxicity, and reach a new equilibrium of health. Homeopathy is like using a thief to catch a thief.

The placebo method is vastly different from the other two kinds of medicine. Placebo is mind over matter. Doctors admit that a placebo is successful most of the time. Medical researchers conduct double-blind studies to prove the effectiveness of a new medication. Some test subjects receive the new drug while some receive a placebo, which is no drug at all. Often, the placebo works as good as, or better than the drug. Adano taught us that the placebo method is successful 99.9 percent of the time.

Placebo's effect starts with our mouths. What comes out of our mouths is just as important as what goes into it, for our CELLS remember everything we say. Have you ever said something and been amazed when it happens? It happens because thoughts are things. Thoughts are also beings. Furthermore, a thought is eternal until it is released.

Speaking and thinking activate a cosmic law, the law of attraction. Whenever you think something, the thought immediately attracts its physical equivalent. When things magnetize toward one another, they move at an ever increasing rate. As a result, thoughts create attraction and acceleration. Thoughts give us the ability to do more with less effort.

For example, you have a thought and speak into it. Speaking into your desire puts the law of attraction (magnetism) into motion. The principle is automatic. We can choose to synchronize with it or not, and it works regardless of our belief system. Most of us fail to realize we have a fantastic gift. We can speak into the utmost in life. Just the same, we can hold ourselves back by what we say. The Rabbi Yhshwh, better known as Jesus, knew about the laws of thought, attraction, and acceleration when he said, "It is written, man shall not live by bread alone, but by every word that proceedeth out of the mouth of God." (Matthew 4:4)

"It is written" is a clear declaration of a systematic record of knowledge and techniques that existed before he made his statement. Rabbi Yhshwh did not think this up, he learned this system from one who knew what life was about. But this knowledge was not for the masses. The ancients hid their understanding of this principle in the symbol of the *Ankh*, also called the Crux Anasta or the Handled Cross.

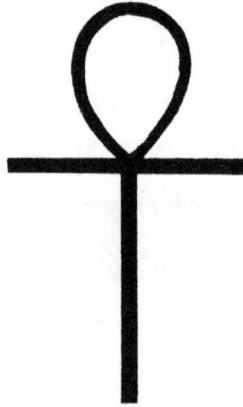

THE ANKH

Historians tell us, the Ankh is the KEY of the Nile. For the masses, it symbolizes health and longevity. To the Initiates of cosmic living, the Ankh embodies the principle of absorbing cosmic Life Energy from the environment and using that Energy to speak into their lives.

The ancients called cosmic Life Energy the "Word of God" because of its audible vibratory rate. The cross of the Ankh represents the body we carry through life. The loop on the top of the Ankh symbolizes the "Mouth of God." Adano taught us, the "Mouth of God" is the medulla oblongata found at the base of our brain.

Scientists tell us the medulla oblongata is the focal point of life. The medulla oblongata traps light like a plant and converts it into cosmic Life Energy in a process similar to photosynthesis. Therefore, light (the sun's radiation) hits the medulla oblongata, is transformed into cosmic Life Energy, and leaves the mouth as BREATH and words.

So we can read Rabbi Yhshwh's (Jesus') statement in more scientific terms as: Man does not live by food alone, but by every word coming from the medulla oblongata as cosmic Life Energy in the breath.

The Rabbi's statement foreshadows man's future development from limited sources of energy (food) to unlimited sources of energy (BREATH).

2. There is a TIME, a PLACE, and a SEASON for EVERYTHING.
—King Solomon, the Solar-man archetype.

The biblical scribe quotes King Solomon saying, "To every thing there is a season, and a time to every purpose under the heaven." (Ecclesiastes 3:1) Adano summarized King Solomon's statements in Ecclesiastes into the second Solar rule:

There is a TIME, a PLACE, and a SEASON for EVERYTHING.

TIME is your health.

PLACE is your pocketbook.

SEASON is your temperature.

TIME

When you spend twenty-thousand dollars for a car, are you buying twenty-thousand dollars worth of parts or twenty-thousand dollars worth of timing? What good is twenty-thousand dollars worth of parts if the car will not run? Timing makes the car run. Similarly, timing keeps our bodies running smoothly. So we can say, TIMING is HEALTH.

TIME TELLS YOU WHAT TO EAT WHEN. You observe how a food grows (in the trees, on a vine, as a root, etc.) and eat it at the peak of its light cycle. TIME is the primary consideration when you decide what to eat. Eating foods in their right time frame gives you the maximum amount of LIGHT from the foods. So we call it eating Solar, or eating LIGHT.

Solar eating resets the human biological clock for maximum assimilation and super immunity. Your CELLS align with Nature. The ancients were students of Nature. They were objective, observant, and discriminating. Their maxim was, "Know Thyself." The ancients used symbols to pass their knowledge to the Initiates of the Sacred Mysteries. Symbolism hid ancient knowledge from the masses and offered a language to embody Nature's purpose.

The most sacred symbol in Egyptian mythology was the beetle, the scarab called *Khepri*. The Egyptians worshipped Khepri as their most potent solar symbol. Egyptian mythology saw Khepri as the image of the self-renewing sun, the god who returns. The sun sets in the evening (dies) and returns in the morning (reborn). Therefore, Khepri symbolized the sun's daily cycle of death and resurrection.

The Egyptians recognized the dung beetle, or scarab, as Nature's model for Khepri on Earth. The dung beetle is not conceived by a female, it produces parthenogenetically—a self-created life. To the Egyptians, Khepri symbolized our ability to self-generate a diamond body from our carbon body.

Furthermore, the dung beetle's larvae develops in the excrement of animals. The Egyptians knew that our excrement determines if we can live like the scarab and have a self-generated resurrection into a new life, or die in our own waste. Legend states how Thoth, the god of medicine and science, transformed himself into a long-billed ibis and injected water into his anus. A few priest-magicians observed the sacred bird's behavior and developed a method to clean the intestines using goatskins filled with water. Egyptian Papyri dating back to the 14th century B.C.E. mention the use of enemas for stomach and intestinal problems. They used the divine clyster for practical treatment of disease and for cellular regeneration. The Egyptians understood the relationship between cleanliness and godliness.

Researchers found Khepri's outline on the walls of the Great Pyramid and it puzzled them. They could not decipher the scarab's hidden alchemistic meaning, for the sacred beetle represents the human body's potential to become something new. Contained within the scarab's outline is the KEY to Solar living. The sacred beetle is a graphic representation of the three different light zones in the human body and how they process food. These three light zones form the basis for eating Solar.

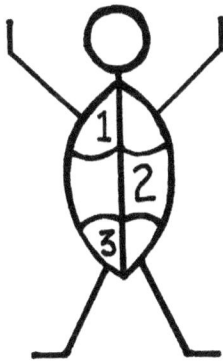

THE SACRED BEETLE
Our Body, Our Spaceship

37

ZONE ONE on the scarab is the 45 degree angle of light, the morning. The foods high up in the trees get the maximum amount of sunlight in the morning. Therefore, we eat fruits and nuts that grow from four feet above the ground and higher between 6 a.m. and 12 noon. We do not heat food in zone one. We eat raw food in the morning. Our bodies secrete the needed enzymes to rapidly digest and completely assimilate morning foods eaten on time.

ZONE TWO on the scarab is the 90 degree angle of light, the afternoon. The leaves on the trees act as an umbrella for fruits and nuts, shielding them from the sun's rays. So we do not eat fruits or nuts from trees in the afternoon. We eat vegetables that grow four inches to four feet above the ground between 12 noon and 6 p.m. These vegetables receive the maximum amount of light at this time of day.

Many vegetables open to absorb the sun's radiation in the 90 degree light range. In zone two, Solar eaters take in grains, two-leggeds, four-leggeds, food from vines, including fruits and vegetables that grow four inches to four feet above the ground. Many of us are the most active during this time frame, so we demand a greater selection of food between 12 noon and 6 p.m. than at other times of day. The 90 degree light range offers the largest variety of foods. Consequently, the midday meal is usually the largest meal of the day. We heat (cook) most of our food in zone two. Also, our bodies produce more digestive secretions during midday than at other times to accommodate the large variety of foods available.

ZONE THREE on the scarab is the bounce light range, the evening. The sun's rays diminish between 6 p.m. and 12 midnight. From 6 p.m. to 9 p.m. Solar eaters ingest foods that grow from four inches above the ground to below the ground like eggs, fish, beets, carrots, mushrooms, and potatoes. Nature did not want us to consume large quantities of food at night. So the variety of foods that grow in the bounce light range (zone three) is small. As with the other light zones, our body secretions match the available food in zone three providing maximum absorption of the nutrients. Also, our bodies produce alcohol at night, which is stored in the spinal column. Evening is the time to use the alcohol in our spinal column as a vehicle for consciousness-raising techniques.

PLACE

The PLACE in King Solomon's statement is the location of your movement; up and down, or back and forth. Location has to do with your pocketbook; the best place to get your pocket food.

Astrocartography is a map of the planets during your birth time and their location on Earth. Adano recommended living under your Jupiter ascending line for the best monetary flow. Money easily flows to you under the influence of beneficial planets. Yet, no matter where you live, eating on time takes priority over location. Thus, Adano insisted, "If you eat on time [Solar eating] you will always be in the right place at the right time and you will never be broke!"

SEASON

The SEASON in King Solomon's statement refers to the body's temperature; a seasonal condition like winter, spring, summer, and fall. Temperature affects the harmony of a relationship, whether it is the relationship of foods in the body, the interaction of two people, or the gravitational pull of two planets. When you take in food on time, the digestive enzymes temperature coincides with the food and you easily burn it. Proper digestion is a seasonal condition, a function of heat and temperature.

Similarly, the season (temperature) is a key factor in harmonious personal relationships. In general, the best match for a man is a woman with the astrological sign that *follows* his on the zodiac wheel. For example, a Leo male is most compatible with a Virgo female. Virgo is an earth sign that helps ground Leo's fire, thus regulating the temperature. Conversely, a woman should be with the astrological sign *before* hers on the zodiac wheel. An Aries woman is most compatible with a Pisces man, because the Pisces man's water will help cool her down so she will not get too hot. If we observe the season, we might have less relationship woes and avoid complaints such as, "She's too hot for me," or "He's a cold fish."

3. Live to EAT to get SICK.

We have 30 years to *muck it up*, and 30 years to clean it up. Thirty years to muck it up means eating without paying attention to timing. Still, we should try to eat healthful food. It stands to reason, if we live on junk food full of chemicals, processed salt, refined sugar, and saturated fats, our health will suffer the consequences—even if we are young. So for the first 30 years of our lives, we can eat whenever we want and the body can handle it. Nature gives us this time to muck it up. Nonetheless, after 30 revolutions around the sun, we cannot handle further abuses without breaking down. Astrologers call it our Saturn return.

Approximately every 30 years Saturn comes around to kick us in the butt and force us to examine our life. Saturn is a strict disciplinarian. It works to help us become more responsible with ourselves. Saturn's influence encourages us to resolve our inner conflicts and clean up previous abuses. Solar eating is a natural way to clean up. Cleaning up takes us from a **who** state, to a **sick** state, to a **What** state in the body. It teaches us how to live to live, rather than living to retire to die.

The persons responsible for you start out as "mom" and "pop" for five minutes in bed. After you are born you call them *parents*, because they pay-the-rent and watch over you for your first 18 years on Earth. Society tells you that you must obey them.

Whether you like it or not, you are stuck with it, until they throw you out to stand on your own.

When the umbilical cord is cut from the mother you become a **who**. Society programs you like programming a computer and tells you how to relate. Over the years you forget **What** you are and accept society's program. You develop a personality, and your personality becomes **who** you are. The word *personality* is derived from the Greek word *persona*, meaning a mask. For most people the mask becomes the person and the individual behind the mask becomes buried under a knot of delusions.

After 18 years—after high school—you have two choices; go to work, or continue your education. You have 12 years to do it before society considers you impractical. For the 12 years from 18 to 30 revolutions around the sun, you are entitled to the joy of mucking it up. No one should deprive you of that. Your first 30 revolutions around the sun are Nature's grace period. If your body is injury free and you stay healthy during this time, you are lucky; count your blessings.

For most of us, the aches and pains start at 30 to 40 revolutions around the sun. So we look for a way to ease our pain. We look to the East and look to the West. If we pay attention, we quickly discover that the answer lies in our CELLS. Nature reminds us that it is time to start cleaning up our act. If we choose not clean it up and continue to muck it up, we choose to fool ourselves, ignore Nature, and avoid **What** we are. Sadly, most of us wait too long before deciding to clean it up and miss our opportunity.

42

At 30 to 40 revolutions around the sun, Saturn's return urges us to come to terms with life. Is it really worth living? Every day we drive down the highway trying to keep up with traffic, hustle at work, and jostle more traffic on the way home. After a while of this exhausting routine, we start to question how practical it is to keep up with society. Once we settle down to sleep, we worry and wonder how we will pay our bills tomorrow. Most of us live this agony every night. And before we finally drift off to sleep, we program our brains to wake up the next day and go to work to pay our bills.

In the morning, we forget everything we said to ourselves the night before, and start the rat race over again. We get up, go to work, pay bills, fight traffic, make more money, increase our spending, to find ourselves deeper in debt. We fear we will not have enough money to pay our bills. Nonetheless, when we get our paycheck, desire (greed) encourages us to spend more than we have. Fear and desire drive us around.

Admittedly, most of us never question beyond our cultural conditioning. If we do question the purpose of life and the dictates of culture, we are considered sick and our friends will recommend a psychiatrist to us. The doctor will put us on powerful tranquilizers and sleeping pills that make sure we never ask those kinds of questions again. Yet deep down inside, we haven't arrived at any acceptance about life. Is this lifestyle really practical? Is life only about eating, sleeping, being merry, having sex, and satisfying our hedonistic desires? Is that what life is about? If so, what is the point?

Moreover, do you know **who** you are, if you are a man or a woman, when you are sound asleep? And what happens if you do not wake up? They will bury you six feet under! You will get the peace society gives, "the peace that passeth all understanding." (Philippians 4:7) They will bury you in your own piece of earth. If you don't wake up before they bury you, you will find your body lying in the grave, and you still will not know **What** you are, because you lost conscious awareness when you fell asleep—you fell asleep on the job. You do not understand what Is happening, because you have not come to terms with **who** you think you are and **What** you actually are.

Nonetheless, you might try to keep up with society for 30, 40, 50, 60, or 70 years. Yet deep down, you do not accept living in a carbon-based body. Also, you do not know **who** you are when you are sound asleep. The rich man and the poor man, the wise man and the ignorant man, have the same problem. They do not know **who** they are—whether they are a man or a woman—when they are sound asleep. They have not resolved life's fundamental question: **Who** or **What** am I?

Nature gives us a model for this conflict within us; the moth and the butterfly. The moth symbolizes the personality, or **who** we think we are. What do moths do? They fly into the light and burn up. They think the light is all there is. They come into the world and never question society's program. Eventually, they burn out. A butterfly, on the other hand, synchronizes with the environment,

44

lives a life of the exception to the rule, transforms its squishy earthbound caterpillar body into a spaceship, and travels to worlds undreamed of by the moth. The butterfly is freed while living, what Sanskrit calls *Jivan Mukta*. Butterflies symbolize the individuality, or **What** we are.

We have two natures within us; the personality (the **who**) and the individuality (the **What**). The personality is egocentric, self-interested, and thinks of everything in terms of its own pleasure and personal enjoyment. The individuality is our God-SELF, or **What** we are. Yet our two natures are not really separate. The individuality is always trying to influence the personality, but since the personality is only interested in its own self-importance, it listens only to itself and remains ignorant of the Presence within.

If you ignore **What** you are and identify with the light like the moth, the world will burn you out. The world and everything in it is made of light, an illusion of the senses. If fear and desire drive you around, you run the risk of getting caught up in the fancy flickering lights of the world and the dictates of culture molding your personality. You will die a death unto your own existence. If you are like the butterfly, however, you will work with **What** you are and start to recognize your individuality as sound—a "still, small voice" within (1 Kings 19:12)—not light.

Our aim in life is to reconcile the conflict between the personality and the individuality by allowing the individuality to consume our personality like fire in a dry wheat field. The Diamond

Body Program ignites within our CELLS, and we become the individuality. We merge light and sound within us, and live in light similar to how a fish lives in water. We live in the world, but not of it. Our individuality lives in our diamond body, our time-space vehicle. Diamond lets light through and is strong enough to take It. The light does not consume us as it does the moth; light feeds us.

If you discover **What** you are and become one with It, you can free yourself (your CELLS) from the fear, the panic, and the frustration of living. You can break free from the programming of tradition and culture, because you will realize it is obsolete. If you devote the time from 30 revolutions around the sun to 60 revolutions around the sun to working with **What** you are, cleaning up your CELLS, you can awaken to your true nature. You may discover **What** you are when you are sound asleep and know what it is like to be deeply asleep, yet wide awake.

Eating on time establishes a bond between the personality and the individuality, and they start to work together. When you sin you are out of synchronicity with **What** you are. Synchronous absorption of food is automatic immortality. You can simply eat your way to butterflyhood, or immortality, because you have no sins hanging over your head. If you look back and think you did something sinful, you'll see it was just a lousy decision. We all make good and lousy decisions. We are not punished for our sins, we are punished by them. We punish our CELLS by creating dis-ease, our pathology, which becomes our PATH to understanding. Let go of the past for it is dead and gone. Forgive your CELLS for past abuses and enter a new highway to health. Rabbi Yhshwh, the master of forgiveness, used the Aramaic word *shaw* for forgive. Shaw means to untie. Untie your CELLS from the past. Untie your SELF from the knot of delusions binding you from living in the present. Free your CELLS. Move into the NOW. Live **What** you are and commit to clean up your act.

We are born into this world as soft, squishy caterpillars. For the first 30 years we are entitled to muck it up. Enjoy it. For when Saturn comes by, it challenges us to clean up our acts. If we ignore Saturn's call to transform, continue to eat whatever we want whenever we want, continue to destroy the environment, and continue to deny **What** we are, we will become a moth, attracted to the light of society's program. For a moth is consumed by the very thing it seeks. The illusion of the world, called *Maya* in Sanskrit, consumes the moth and it burns out. The moth lives to eat, to sleep, to be merry, to have sex, to retire, and to die. It ends up in the earth from whence it came.

Meanwhile, life gives us another WAY. If we heed Saturn's reminder to clean it up, start to eat on time all the time, work with the environment, and listen to **What** we are, we may become a beautiful butterfly sustained by sound, living in the light of the world, but not consumed by it. The environment our DNA lives in will change and every CELL in our body could transform into the immortal diamond body.

The answer to life's riddle is in your genetics. You choose to synchronize with It or not. The choice is yours, and yours alone: Moth or Butterfly?

4. Live to EAT NOT to GET SICK.

Most people live to eat, to retire, to get sick, to die. A synchronized life offers another choice. We can eat NOT to get sick. Eating to not get sick involves four steps:

- clean up
- more selective
- less food
- phase out food altogether

The Solar process takes you from eating mostly tissue (meat), to eating mostly fiber (vegetables), to drinking mostly liquid (juices), to getting nourishment from air alone (breatharian).

Adano encouraged us to clean up our acts by eating Solar and promptly eliminating the waste. Most of the time, we need specialized colonics to get rid of residual buildup. If the excess is not removed in a timely fashion, autointoxication results. Robert Gray (1991) in his booklet titled, *The Colon Health Handbook* defines autointoxication on page 15 as:

> ...the process whereby the body literally poisons itself by maintaining a cesspool of decaying matter in its colon. This inner cesspool can contain as high a concentration of harmful bacteria as a cesspool under a house. The toxins released by the decay process get into the

bloodstream and travel to all parts of the body. Every cell in the body gets affected, and many forms of sickness can result. Because it weakens the entire system, autointoxication can be a causative factor for nearly any disease.

We call Adano's specialized colonics *hydropathy*, meaning "the empirical use of water in the treatment of disease." (Webster's Ninth New Collegiate Dictionary) Dis-ease is any disorder in the body.

Adano's hydropathic device is an inspired design for a thorough evacuation. Hydropathy gives a completely different mental and emotional experience from the traditional type of colonic. A regular colonic is a closed system. Water is injected into the large intestine where it is held unnaturally and mechanically released. Hydropathy, on the other hand, uses an open system to allow the body's own rhythm to cleanse its CELLS. Warm gravity-fed, purified water enters the large intestine and releases without holding or straining. The body determines for itself how to best use the water. In a sense, your body treats itself, and given a chance, will clean its CELLS in short order.

By analogy, hydropathy is like lying on warm sand on a tropical beach with your feet pointing toward the ocean. Warm water gently washes up your legs to your midsection and recedes. As each wave tenderly washes over you, your mind releases stored trauma and your thinking clears. The ocean water carries your traumas out to the sea and cleanses them. Hydropathy works exactly like warm ocean waves inside your body. Water purifies you from the inside out.

Adano said, "Cleanliness is Godliness, dirtiness is death."

The great Bulgarian philosopher and spiritual Master, Omraam Mikhael Aivanhov (1900-1986), emigrated to France in 1937, where he lived and taught for almost 50 years. Mr. Aivanhov talked about "cleaning up" in alchemistic terms:

> As long as human beings stay outside of God, they do not know Him. In order to understand the immensity of God we must merge with Him, lose ourselves in Him, fuse with Him. But this fusion cannot occur unless we work at purifying ourselves. Let us use the image of a large drop of mercury: you spread it in tiny droplets over a sheet of paper and then form one big drop again. You have no doubt all carried out this experiment. Now sprinkle some dust on the tiny droplets spread out all over the sheet of paper. Whatever you do to bring them back together again, they remain separate. Well, this is what happens with us. The Lord is splendor, light, immensity, and to come closer to Him we must eliminate all these impurities which, like the dust, prevent fusion from taking place. (Prosveta, p.251, *Daily Meditations*, 1999)

If we want to merge with God, or **What** we are, we purify our CELLS, or clean up our acts. Adano's cleaning up program is twofold:

1)eat Solar

2)clean out the waste

Eating Solar is a rapid detoxification of the mechanism. If you pile up all the toxins released when you eat Solar on top of years of accumulated waste, autointoxication is almost guaranteed. Therefore, Adano recommended a *series* of hydropathy sessions to clean out the colon. A series is a 10 week program of 12 colon lavages. The first two weeks you have two sessions per week. Then you have one session a week for the next eight weeks. For most people, a series will allow water to flow through the entire length of the large intestine. Then you continue hydropathy as needed.

We should strive to clean up our colons. The health of the entire body depends on the health of the colon. Constipation is the number one affliction underlying nearly every ailment. Yet, health authorities almost ignore the most common condition afflicting the mass of humanity on Earth. Nearly every person living in modern society today is constipated whether they know it or not. The condition is so common that medical authorities consider constipation normal!

Your body is the house God lives in. It stands to reason, the building you make your home needs periodic cleaning. If you left the kitchen garbage lying around and never emptied it, your house would stink. Essentially, your colon is the same as a trash can. Your colon stores the waste products of metabolism and digestion for elimination. If your colon is not evacuated in a timely fashion, the resulting condition is similar to neglecting to take out the kitchen garbage. The waste in your colon putrefies, decays, and generates gas and toxic substances. Putrefaction causes autointoxication in the intestinal tract. Toxins release into your bloodstream and poison your entire system. Your immunity is compromised and sickness is often the result.

As was mentioned, five million cells die and five million cells are reborn each second. Every forty days your body replaces all its minerals. Every seven years your body replaces all its cells. The magnetic push (dilation) and pull (constriction) of the body is called *metabolism*. Metabolism has two basic phases:

> …*anabolism*, the constructive phase, during which small molecules resulting from the digestive process are built up into complex compounds that form the tissues and organs of the body; and *catabolism* the destructive phase, during which larger molecules are broken down into simpler substances with the release of energy. (*Barron's Dictionary of Medical Terms*, second ed., 1989)

Broken down tissue is toxic. Toxins are a by-product of metabolism, as constant and necessary as life.

In a healthy body, the blood and lymph collect and eliminate the metabolic waste matter from everywhere in the system. This waste does not poison us, because our body uses *nerve-energy* to remove the debris as fast as it is produced. When nerve-energy is squandered, the body becomes *enervated*. Enervation slows the removal of metabolism's residue. When elimination is incomplete, the blood and organs retain toxins. If metabolic waste-products overwhelm the body, *Toxemia* results.

J. H. Tilden, M.D. (1851-1940), the son of a physician, practiced medicine his entire life. As a young doctor, he became disillusioned with medical practice and resolved to quit the profession or find the cause of disease. Dr. Tilden found that retention of metabolic toxins, what he called Toxemia, is the first and only cause of disease. Dr. Tilden concluded; only Nature cures. Consequently, he maintained that there are no medical cures for disease and that diagnosis is a "medical delusion." (p.93) Nature insists we clean up our acts, or else!

Eating out of time and emotions such as shock, grief, anger, envy, gossiping, selfishness, ambition, jealousy, dishonesty, egotism, self-indulgence, and business worries enervate the body. Dr. Tilden identifies fear as "the greatest of all causes of enervation." (p.108) Fear is misunderstanding life and its purpose. We have nothing to fear, yet the memory of past failures keeps fear alive. We forget that the initiator of our actions is the one God within us. When we doubt that God will take care of our needs, fear controls us and feeds the ego's vampiric desires. Yet all our experiences in life, good and bad, polish the diamond in the rough and should not be judged.

Fear controls us by drawing what we fear to us. Look at how our CELLS function. Our mechanism works like an electromagnet.

Trace minerals give us primarily electrical qualities. Basic minerals give us primarily magnetic qualities. Yet all minerals are electromagnetic to some degree except iron and carbon. An electromagnet has an iron core. Similarly, we have an iron and carbon core. Iron is the most important element in the blood and it operates by magnetic pressure, not electronically. The iron core of an electromagnet is wrapped with coils of wire through which passes an electric current. Electric current also passes through the minerals in our system. The stronger the electrical current, the stronger the magnetic field. A strong magnetic field creates concentrated lines of flux that pull objects close to the core.

Furthermore, the strength of an electromagnet amplifies with the number of times the wire is wound around the core. For example, vibrations of fear are strong electrical impulses that magnetically draw to a person the fear of others. Each time we dwell on the idea feared, we wrap another wire around the core of our being and magnetically strengthen the fearful idea. With enough reinforcement, the idea feared is magnetically drawn into our orbit and becomes reality.

Worry is the second greatest cause of enervation and is an outgrowth of fear. Because you magnetically attract what you think about, worry is like succeeding in reverse. Studies show that 40 percent of people's worries are about things that will never happen, 30 percent of people's worries are about things that have already happened, 12 percent of people's worries are about health, 10 percent of people's worries are about petty miscellaneous things, and only 8 percent of people's worries are legitimate.

British statesman and author Winston Churchill (1874-1965) said, "When I look back on all these worries, I remember the story of the old man who said on his deathbed that he had a lot of trouble in his life, most of which never happened."

Adano said simply, "Worry kills."

Life is 50/50: Fifty percent positive and fifty percent negative. Nothing in the universe, in the long-run, is just one way. Ancient Chinese philosophers called it Yin/Yang. Day follows night, spring follows winter, victory follows defeat, and success follows failure. Losing is a part of winning and making mistakes is a part of succeeding. Forgive yourself for the mistakes you made. Learn from the past, do not live in the past. Focus all your energies on the present moment and what you plan to do in the future. Remember: Keep trying, because you can't lose 'em all!

We can believe all our lives we are losers, but scientific facts prove us wrong. Whether we are male or female, we are the combination of a sperm and an ovum. The sperm that made it to the ovum to become you won the race up the uterine canal. The hardy sperm, which is half of what you are, is a winner. The ovum accepted the best swimmer and became a winner itself. Everyone born through the birth canal is a winner, because losers can't be born. Thus science proves, we are all winners. Furthermore, as long as you keep breathing day after day, you are on top of the journey to **What** you are. BREATH sustains us. As long as we breathe, we have nothing to worry about.

Indian nationalist and spiritual leader Mahatma Gandhi (1869-1948) said it best, "There is nothing that wastes the body like worry, and one who has any faith in God should be ashamed to worry about anything whatsoever."

We are here to overcome what we say and finish it, so we will not have to come back and do it over. Cleaning up the body and purifying the brain is the first step to facing **What** you are and discovering the principle of HEALTH living within your CELLS. Eating on time (eating Solar) is automatic self-cleaning. Also, eating Solar creates a profound change in behavior. That is the important point. We start to recognize our enervating habits and work with them.

Adano said, "Time does not heal, timing does."

As explained in the second Solar rule, timing determines our health. Timing is *when* we eat, not necessarily what we eat. Eating on time is a natural self-cleaning, self-regenerating process. Adano's way to health agrees with Dr. Tilden's Philosophy of Toxemia, because they understand that time does not cure disease, Nature does.

Furthermore, eating food out of time and emotionally enervating habits build every disease in the mind and body. Dr. Tilden sums it up in the preface of *Toxemia Explained* (Health Research, 1981) as follows:

> From time immemorial, man has looked for a savior; and, when not looking for a savior, he is looking for a cure. He

believes in paternalism. He is looking to get something for nothing, not knowing that the highest price we ever pay for anything is to have it given to us.

Instead of accepting salvation, it is better to deserve it. Instead of buying, begging, or stealing a cure, it is better to stop building disease. Disease is of man's own building, and one worse thing than the stupidity of buying a cure is to remain so ignorant as to believe in cures.

The false theories of salvation and cures have built man into a mental mendicant, when he should be the arbiter of his own salvation, and certainly his own doctor, instead of being a slave to a profession that has neither worked out its own salvation from disease nor discovered a single cure in all the age-long period of man's existence on earth. (p.9)

Law and order drive the universe. When we live in accord with Nature, health automatically happens. As we start to clean up our acts and eat on time, we synchronize with the environment. Removing toxic buildup from the body gives the system a chance to cleanse its CELLS physically and mentally. Hydropathy contributes to clearing the trauma contained within the CELLS without the need for psychoanalysis. Yet, hydropathy is only a portion of the equation for HEALTH. The other part is eating Solar. They work hand-in-hand for cellular regeneration and transformation. God is pure HEALTH; not something you buy in a store, but a wonderful Principle flowing within you.

The Solar eater is involved with a something for something lifestyle, not something for nothing consciousness. We start with food, because eating is a way to maintain or change behavior. Eating Solar is a metamorphic lifestyle, not a diet. We eat on time and wait for change to come from within our structure. Hence, waiting is the highest science. While we wait, we avoid four things at *all times* for our health. Stay away from:

1) **Popcorn**: The hard kernel is indigestible. It can cling to the intestinal wall causing irritation and adding to retention in that area. The lodged kernel can create an irritation on the intestinal wall, leading to infection.

2) **Melted cheese**: The chemical reaction of heating cheese creates an indigestible plastic with a high amount of lactic acid (mucous) content that clogs your intestines.

3) **Deep fried foods**: Frying food creates a coating similar to varnish that is difficult to digest, so it accumulates in the large intestine. Heating oil alters the fat molecules that lead to arteriosclerosis or build-up of plaque in the arteries. In addition, deep fried foods are the main cause of gallstones.

4) **Carbonated Fluids**: Each American drinks approximately 50 gallons of soft drinks a year. Most soft drinks contain carbonated fluid with large amounts of refined sugar. Drinking carbonated fluids upsets the calcium-phosphorus balance in the body, thus interfering with calcium absorption. Carbonated drinks add carbon dioxide to your system, which rob you of vital oxygen and escalate bone

deterioration. If you drink carbonated beverages daily it can cause rickets, osteoporosis, rheumatoid arthritis, and a host of other degenerative diseases. Carbon dioxide storage bloats the stomach. Furthermore, carbon dioxide can cause a fat cell to expand more than 1,000 times its original size. Iced drinks are one of the worst things for our bodies. Cold drinks cause the tiny fibers lining the walls of the small intestines, called the *villi*, to contract. When the villi contract, digestion is impaired. Foods eaten with cold drinks are not efficiently metabolized and are stored in fat for use later. Thus drinking cold drinks contributes to weight gain and carbon dioxide retention. We release trapped carbon dioxide by yawning, groaning, yelling, sighing, burping, and farting.

LUNAR EATING

Solar eating gives the body a rapid clean out. Yet sometimes the detoxification is too fast. So each month we practice Lunar eating, or potluck eating. We still avoid four things; popcorn, deep fried, melted cheese, and carbonated drinks, because they don't digest well anytime. During the Lunar cycle, we can eat most anything (except the four things) at anytime without harming our system. We call it Lunar eating, because we do it at the time of the full moon.

As the moon exerts pressure on the tides, it puts pressure on our bodies. Full moon cycle is a natural pressure cycle for better eliminations. Foods eaten out of time will move on through and not constipate you during the full moon period. Also, Lunar eating makes our system work harder than when we eat Solar, thus increasing our immunity. Lunar eating allows us to "be in the world but not of it." (Blum, p.63, The Book of Runes, St. Martin's Press, 1982)

Your body is the car you drive through life. The food you put into your mouth is the gas and oil that fuels your body/car. Foods eaten on time are high octane fuels. An engine burns high octane fuel more efficiently with less toxic emissions. Similarly, the body/car metabolizes and eliminates food eaten on time easier than foods eaten out of time. Solar eating gives your body/car high octane fuel which acts as an accelerator; a rapid detoxification and mechanism decarbonization.

Still, you do not want to go too fast. If you go too fast, you might lose control, crash, and burn. Nature gives us Lunar eating to decelerate. Lunar eating is akin to a car's brakes against the wheels. It allows you to control the speed of acceleration by slowing down detoxification. Lunar eating is a temporary braking system to regulate the speed of clean up. Also, it is Nature's way to break the monotony. So, eat Solar most of the time and take a break each full moon to eat Lunar.

We can free our CELLS from self-destructive habits by reassigning the time we eat food. As a result, we develop more compassion for ourselves and for others on the road of life.

For the first 30 years you practice potluck eating, or Lunar eating. When the aches and pains come on around 30 to 40 years, you need to clean up your act or your body/car will start to breakdown. If you eat out of time (Lunar), all the time, you will be out of time mechanically. Being out of time mechanically means you lack environmental synchronicity. Life will be a rough road.

Potluck eating during Solar time leads to a breakdown of the mechanism, akin to using low octane gas in a car when it needs high octane. If you eat on time and clean up your mechanism, you give your body/car high octane fuel, which give your CELLS the energy to go from a **sick** state to a **What** state within your mechanism. The journey is; from a **who** state, to a **sick** state, to a **What** state within your body.

Until you are ready to take full charge of your health, you remain sick. Thus, your pathology becomes your PATH through life. You create it as an opportunity to progress in your understanding. When faced with your pathology (your PATH) you make a conscious choice to live or to die. Consequently, all death is suicide. If you choose to die, you will see death is simply a change in a way of life, a *cosmic vacation.*

Everything goes through cycles of change. Many researchers (Robert A. Monroe, Kenneth Ring, Dannion Brinkley, Betty J. Eadie, Raymond Moody, M.D., and others) have proved beyond a shadow of a doubt that we survive a decent burial. Death is a fiction, a game we play with our nonexistent selves. What we call death is the end of one form and the birth of another. Nothing *goes* anywhere, energy simply changes form.

Trees lose their leaves in the fall and when spring arrives, new leaves grow. A maple tree is still alive when it has no leaves in the middle of winter. Similarly, perennial flowers die each winter and shrivel, yet they grow again in the spring. Birds lose their feathers when they molt, but they still fly. New feathers grow to replace the old. Animals lose their thick winter fur and grow lighter fur in the warm time of year. Changing one form to another is the natural cycle of life. Everything changes.

When we go on cosmic vacation we shed our physical body like a snake shedding its skin. We abandon the skin of our earthy bodies and return to the holographic projection of our physical self. Our holographic projection continues to live in subspace with other holographic selves until it finds another physical body to live in.

After our cosmic vacation, we get a new chemical body to work with. We call it reincarnation. The ancients called it the Wheel of Life. No matter how you label it, the fact remains, death is an illusion. Death is a change in LIFE, and LIFE is everlasting. We do not go anywhere, because there is no where to go except HERE and NOW.

Yet you have free choice, and there are no wrong choices. You cannot choose the wrong road, because there is no way out of life! You can, however, take the direct road or the delay road. If you take the delay road, you choose to remain sick. If you take the direct road, you choose to live to eat not to get sick. In other words, you choose to eat Solar. Eating Solar is the direct road, because you surrender your willpower to its Higher Nature. This willpower is directed from without, or "Thy will be done."

The decision to work with your environment, walk your PATH within your pathology and learn from it, brings you to the final step in the Solar process; discovering **What** you are.

5. LIVE TO EAT in order to LIVE *NOT* TO EAT (MEMORY PATTERN).

The person who knows **What** they are is a diamond body individual, a permanent fixture in the universe. The veils of ignorance and illusion are gone. The ever-present ME surrounds and sustains them day and night. The person who knows **What** they are doesn't need to eat or sleep anymore.

The diamond body individual is more common than you might think. World religions, much literature, and many personal life experiences contain interactions with diamond body individuals. For example, Robert A. Monroe (1915-1995) founder of the Monroe Institute, achieved worldwide recognition as a groundbreaking visionary and explorer of human consciousness. In his book, *Ultimate Journey* (Doubleday, 1994) Mr. Monroe contacts the "most mature and evolved human in physical earth" living in current time. (p.50) He called the person a "true equal—a He/She." (p.51) Mr. Monroe stated that He/She has lived for eighteen hundred years and gave up eating and sleeping "years ago." (p.53)

He/She is one of many diamond body mechanisms who remains in the physical. Most diamond body types live in subspace and manifest in the physical when they choose. Once you reach the diamond body state, the choice to remain in the physical body or live in the subspace realm is yours. A diamond body person can appear or disappear at will. Whether in the physical body full-time or not, the diamond body person drops their addiction to eating and sleeping when they become the end-product of human evolution. Eating Solar conditions the body to live on less and less food until it switches to living on air alone.

We can get to the non-eating state by fasting, injury, a genetic condition, or the natural way. Fasting is an internal decision. Sometimes you make it, sometimes you don't. Injury, however, is forced upon you from without. Sometimes after an injury or a genetic condition, the body might not be able to handle food and you phase out eating. Fasting, injury, or a genetic condition are valid approaches to the non-eating state.

Yet cosmic Intelligence set up a natural way, what the biblical scribe called "threescore and ten." (Psalms 90:10) "Threescore and ten" means 60 to 70 revolutions around the sun, the innate cycle for the body's switchover to the non-eating state. At "threescore and ten" we need less food, less sleep, and our bodies go through a profound change. We absorb more vitality from light and air. If we have cleaned up our acts between 30 and 60 revolutions, around 60 to 70 revolutions we can quit eating with our mouths and start living with our nose. We may automatically shift to a diamond body, like a car shifting gears to run at a higher speed.

Our carbon-based body has 144 elements; 108 functional minerals and 36 radicals to harass you. The elements in your body can vibrate at different speeds. At one speed your CELLS can vibrate with the ego, the personality. At another speed your CELLS can vibrate with your inherited individual rhythm, your God-SELF, the diamond-based body. When your body shifts to the rhythm of the individuality at 60 to 70 revolutions, you can become a living model of resurrection in a carbon body, a living example of "not my will, but Thy Will be done." You can master the carbon frame simply by vibrating at a different rate. Above all, it helps if you have conditioned your system to handle it.

When you master a carbon-based body, you vibrate as an individuality with the rhythm of the universe as One. You are in tune with cosmic Will. What sustains you in that state of being is not food or sleep, but cosmic Energy as BREATH. Your CELLS resurrect into an immortal, indestructible mechanism, maintained by BREATH as light and sound.

In addition, your chakra system becomes a fully functional wave-guide for cosmic rays. Sunlight and starlight are primary light, with moonlight being reflected sunlight. The chakras and human aura refract light and sound into levels of bio-electricity. Bio-electricity from cosmic radiation sustains the diamond body mechanism while oxygen (BREATH) gives it consciousness. You no longer live by processing food through eating and elimination, you live by processing light directly from the Source. Because light does not decompose, immortality of the human mechanism is possible.

Thus, your carbon-based body can resurrect into a diamond-based body, a permanent fixture in the universe. Resurrection is the final journey in the Solar process. The resurrected person knows, without any doubt, **What** they are.

Radiance (light) and Sonics (sound) run the show. There is nothing here but light and sound playing the charade of eating and sleeping. **What** you are is a unique combination of 144 elements (called a BODY) functioning as the atomic structure of the universe. God (Sonics) slipped into you through your mouth as BREATH. Because you breathe, you are conscious and can relate to the world. If you keep breathing, you have the opportunity to be here NOW and realize **What** you are.

BREATH provides equality, not superiority. When it comes to the BREATH we are all the same. BREATH is equally available all around. But when you think you are special, equality can be hard to live with.

BREATH also gives us the opportunity to speak. So our mouths become our best friend and our worst enemy. Every word we say and think is manifested within the atomic structure of creation, because we are one with It. We create our own reality. Therefore, we must live what we say and finish it.

God is a cosmic Principle flowing through us as BREATH with no beginning or end.

Adano defined God as, "LOVE in the form of gas working through vegetation." LOVE is magnetism; an attraction and repulsion, a constriction and dilation. The four gases working through the carbon-based body are:

> **1) Hydrogen.** Your body uses hydrogen to regulate and generate desire in you, a constriction and dilation process.

68

Desire stimulates belief. *De* means dual. *Sire* means rule, reproduce yourself, and Xerox yourself. Thus, de-sire (hydrogen) regulates your sex drive. Also hydrogen produces the desire to act, which regulates your belief in yourself. Metabolically, hydrogen breaks down protein.

2) Nitrogen. We need nitrogen to live. Nitrogen regulates willpower. Willpower (nitrogen) is desire (hydrogen) plus energy (sunlight). Willpower can be directed inward or outward. Inward directed willpower is "my will be done." Outward directed willpower is "Thy will be done." Raw foods contain abundant nitrogen. Adano taught us that if you eat protein without nitrogen (raw food), it will cause cancer. He also told us that if you eat protein plus nitrogen (raw food), it will prevent cancer. Adano defined cancer as, "Dogmatic bullheadedness wanting to prove it is never wrong—possessiveness by lashing out." If a lump appears, he recommended eating lots of protein with nitrogen (raw) foods. A healthy balance for most people is 80 percent raw, 20 percent cooked.

3) Oxygen. Oxygen produces the phenomenon called consciousness, which is the Breath of Life, not the intellect. Consciousness is a camera-izing effect, a photographic condition. When oxygen entered the nose with the first breath, it hit the pituitary gland, thus regulating the lungs and bodily functions. Scientists call this the "resonance factor." Resonance is the intensity or power of God residing in the geometry (flesh).

4) Carbon Dioxide. Carbon dioxide is a waste gas created by burning the other three gases and solids during metabolism. Fatigue is over-retention of carbon dioxide in the system. Carbon dioxide has two functions; destructive and constructive. Too much carbon dioxide will kill you. A little carbon dioxide will refrigerate (preserve) you forever.

Now we can understand Adano's definition of God as LOVE (a magnetic constricting and dilating condition) in the form of gas (hydrogen, nitrogen, oxygen, and carbon dioxide) working through vegetation (human flesh and the environment). Given this definition, God is ever-present as YOU. God is not some person sitting on a throne in a sterile corner of the universe waiting to judge dead people. God is YOU. You can tell yourself that you live to die, or you live to retire to die. But when you finally go on cosmic vacation you will be disappointed, because God is not there waiting for you. God waits for no one. God is LIFE living here and now as BREATH within the geometry of human flesh. All life is action. So God is LIFE as ACTION in the here and now. God is of the living, not of the dead. Even Rabbi Yhshwh said, "He is not the God of the dead, but the God of the living." (Mark 12:27)

Faced with the scientific facts of God living in the human mechanism as LOVE in the form of four gases can be hard to accept in light of cultural conditioning. Letting go of childhood programming can be a challenge. Paul said, "When I was a child, I spake as a child, I understood as a child, I thought as a child: but when I became a man, I put away childish things." (1 Corinthians 13:11) Paul came to the point in his life where he had to let go of his cultural beliefs to accept the facts of **What** he was.

Society programs us to believe many childish myths. Unless we can let go of our treasured childhood beliefs, we will not discover the facts behind the myths. As adults, life challenges us to face the facts of **What** we are and let go of **who** we think we are. Life constantly puts before us the truth of our divine nature, but cultural myths block our view. Let me share some childhood myths I let go of when I became a man and matured in understanding.

When I was a child I believed Santa Claus was a real person. I thought he lived in a place called the North Pole. I pictured his pudgy frame with rosy cheeks, a wavy white beard, in a red suit with white fur trim, driving a sleigh full of presents pulled by famous reindeer. I saw him on television and dreamed about him Christmas eve. I believed Santa Claus gave all the good children presents and did not give presents to those who were bad. I tried to be a very good boy. Yet when I became a man, I bought what I needed and what I wanted at Christmas time. I bought gifts for my loved ones and put the presents under the tree on Christmas morning. When I matured in understanding, I realized, I was Santa Claus.

Similarly, when I was a child I believed Uncle Sam was a real person. I thought he was a thin, old, kindly gentleman who worked for the government. I saw his smiling face on posters and on television. He stood outside government offices on tax day waving and smiling. He wore red and white striped pants, a blue tailcoat, and a blue top hat with white stars on the brim. Yet, when I became a man and began to work and pay taxes, I saw how my taxes supported the government. I realized that Uncle Sam did not work for the government, I did. When I matured in understanding, I realized, I was Uncle Sam.

Furthermore, when I was a child in Sunday school they taught me about God. They showed me pictures of Him sitting like a judge and king on a throne. I envisioned his stern face behind a long gray beard, living in a sterile corner of the universe called Heaven, a place protected by pearly gates. Saint Peter sat in the security guard shack outside Heaven's gate and checked the names on his clipboard to see who would get in. The church authorities told me, "God will reward you if you are good and He will punish you if you are bad." For God sat in Heaven and would judge me when I died. Yet when I became a man, I learned through trial and error, that I was the one who punished or rewarded myself by my thoughts, words, and actions. Consequently, I judged myself, right here, right now. I learned that I was the only God there ever was or ever will be. I understood that God is everything, all creation. Not only does God live inside me as a divine Spark, my body lives inside the body of God. When I matured in understanding, I realized, I was God.

Tradition programmed into my imagination the myths of Santa Claus, Uncle Sam, and God. I had to see the fallacy of these childhood myths before I could free myself from their bondage. Paul admonished the Gelatins saying, "…as long as he is a child, [he] differs nothing from a servant, though he be Lord of all." (Galatians 4:1)

You are Lord of all. **What** you are is God—not a person sitting on a throne in heavenly heights—but a cosmic Principle that offers the opportunity to talk to its SELF in a human body. This cosmic Principle (God) gives us every possible test from sleep, to memory, to forgetfulness. God asks us to rise above these challenges and remember **What** we are.

Men and women are subject to the laws of Nature when they live in a carbon-based body on Earth. As long as we remain ignorant of Nature's law, we will be subject to the Law. When we begin working with the five Solar rules, we throw off ignorance—the ignoring principle—and start to understand how life functions. The minute we understand the nature of the Law, it becomes subject to us. We rise above our limitations and discover **What** we are. When we understand that God is in us, God becomes subject to us, and becomes our servant. We discover that we don't work for God, God works for us.

So when you know **What** you are when you are sound asleep and can get up and live without sleeping anymore, you have found what all the great saints and sages of the world know: You and the creative Life are One and the same. Gone are the veils of ignorance, illusion, and imagination. The ever-present I AM surrounds you, day or night, eyes open or eyes closed.

When you know **What** you are, Solar eating ends and a new life begins. You resurrect from a carbon body type to a diamond body type as the caterpillar becomes the butterfly. Your CELLS unite with God and become indestructible, incorruptible, immortal, as God is immortal. The diamond body is yours forever. You receive your cosmic Oscar for a performance well done. Your new body absorbs cosmic Life Energy directly from the environment. You no longer need to take in energy indirectly as food in the form of solids and liquids. Eating is obsolete for the diamond body person, because cosmic Life Energy in BREATH as light and sound support you.

We can live two ways in this world. When you are a child, you have a something for nothing attitude. Momma and Poppa give you what you need to survive as long as you obey them. When you grow up the world tells you, "Hey fella, this is a something for something world." You will not continue to get something for nothing, so do not fool yourself for too long.

Enjoy your childhood days. You are entitled to it. Yet remember: When you mature, life is something for something. The choice between a something for nothing lifestyle or a something for something lifestyle is up to you.

HOW TO EAT YOUR MEDITATION
General Guidelines

THE ALMOND

Of all the nuts, the almond is king. The word *almond* is French for *all world*. Almonds are the only food containing all twelve basic minerals. Our bodies are mineral processors and almonds nourish our mechanisms with more basic minerals than any other food. Thus, the almond is the king of foods.

Edgar Cayce (1877–1945) the clairvoyant known as the sleeping prophet, went into a trance state twice a day and contacted Universal consciousness. He provided medical suggestions to thousands of people who requested readings. Sandra Duggan, R.N. writes in her book *Edgar Cayce's Guide to Colon Care* (1995), "If two to three raw almonds with the brown skins intact are taken daily as a snack or properly combined with other food, Cayce said we never need fear cancer." (p.57) Sandra Duggan quotes Mr. Cayce:

> An almond a day is much more in accord with keeping the doctor away, especially certain types of doctors, than apples. For the apple was the fall, not the almond–for the almond blossomed when everything else died. Remember this is life! (p.57)

Almonds should be uncooked and presoaked. Leave the skin on, for it has many beneficial properties. Soak your almonds in distilled water a minimum of six hours, and no longer than three days. Keep them refrigerated for freshness.

The first bite of the day should be an almond to set the full strength of your stomach's hydrochloric acid for all day protein digestion. Adano recommended eating one presoaked almond for every ten pounds of functional body weight. (For example, if your functional weight is 120 pounds, eat 12 soaked almonds each morning.)

REHYDRATE

Whenever you eat dried fruit or nuts, rehydrate them first. Rinse them in tap water, drain it off, and then cover them with distilled water. Let them soak at least overnight and always refrigerate them. If you eat dried foods without replacing their liquid before ingestion, they are more difficult to digest and will dehydrate you.

COBALAMIN SYRUP
(One cup a day minimum, two cups maximum)

Morning coffee consists of one cup of mountain grown organic coffee with one teaspoon of pure organic cocoa and the darker type (grade B) pure maple syrup to taste.

Adano called this brew *cobalamin syrup,* a hormone balancer. Another name for cobalamin is vitamin B-12, which alleviates stress, fatigue, and depression. A morning cup of cobalamin syrup removes the excess carbon dioxide accumulated during sleep, boosts energy and mental concentration, strengthens skeletal muscles, and stimulates the kidneys and large intestines for more efficient elimination.

FIVE ELEMENTS

A complete meal has five elements to encourage digestion: 1)Protein, 2)Carbohydrates, 3)Oils, 4)Liquids, 5)Vitamins and Minerals

ZONE ONE: Dawn to 12 noon

BREAKFAST (Dawn to 10 a.m.): Eat foods that grow from four feet above the ground to foods that grow high on trees.

    1)Protein (nuts): Almonds, Brazil nuts, Carob, Cashews, Filberts, Pecans, Pinon, Pistachio, Walnuts

    2)Carbohydrates (fruits): Apples, Apricots, Bananas (after you peel the banana, shave off the outer starchy layer with a dull knife to help it digest easier), Cherries, Dates, Figs, Mangoes, Nectarines, Olives, Peaches, Pears, Papaya, Persimmons, Prunes

    3)Oils (1 to 2 tablespoons on food or by mouth): Use only organic cold-pressed oils such as Almond oil, Apricot oil, Avocado oil, Olive oil, or Walnut oil.

    4)Liquids (juices): Apple, Apricot, Peach, Pear, Papaya

    5)Vitamins and Minerals (derived from the above foods)

MID-MORNING SNACK (10 a.m.): This time is for citrus fruits. Eat citrus fruits *alone*. Eat nothing one hour before or one hour after eating them, as they do not combine well with other foods. Citrus fruits include oranges, grapefruits, lemons, limes, and tangerines (also their fresh squeezed juices).

In ZONE ONE, *always cook* cashews and coconut.

ZONE TWO: 12 noon to 6 p.m.

LUNCH (12 noon to 4 p.m.): Eat foods that grow from four inches above the ground to four feet above ground.

1)Protein (high quality meats and seeds): Beef, Buffalo, Fowl, Lamb, Pork, Venison; Chia seeds, Flax seeds, Poppy seeds, Pumpkin seeds, Sesame seeds, Sunflower seeds

2)Carbohydrates (grains, vegetables): Barley, Beans, Bell Pepper, Broccoli, Brussel Sprouts, Cauliflower, Celery tops, Corn, Cucumber, Eggplant, Lettuce, Millet, Oats, Okra, Parsley, Peas, Peppers, Rice, Rye, Spinach, Sprouts, Squash, Tomatoes, Wheat

3)Oil (1 to 2 tablespoons on food or by mouth): Olive Oil, Ghee, Safflower Oil, Sesame Oil, Sunflower Oil, Wheat Germ Oil

4)Liquids (juices): Cranberry, Grape, Spinach, Tomato

5)Vitamins and Minerals (derived from the above foods)

MID-AFTERNOON SNACK (4 p.m.): Melons are a great mid-afternoon snack. Caution: Eat melons *alone*. Eat nothing one hour before or after eating them, as they do not combine well with other foods. Other afternoon snacks include strawberries, grapes, raisins, and blueberries.

Between 3 p.m. and 5 p.m. is a good time for a glass of *red* wine. Red wine gives your body rich antioxidants called *pycnogenols*.

Antioxidants strengthen the immune system and fight off free radicals that attack cells.

Change champagne into *grapede* by adding a little honey and stirring until the bubbles are gone. Cheers!

In ZONE TWO, *always cook* the following foods:

Artichoke leaves

Bell pepper

Eggplant

Rhubarb

Tomatoes (unless vine-ripened)

DO NOT COOK SPINACH

ZONE THREE: 6 p.m. to 9 p.m.

DINNER (6 p.m. to 9 p.m.): Eat foods that grow from four inches above the ground to under the ground and in water (the bounce light range).

1)Protein: Eggs, Fish, Peanuts

2)Carbohydrates (vegetables, rice): Artichoke hearts, Asparagus, Bamboo shoots, Beets, Carrots, Celery root and bottom four inches of the stalk, Garlic, Ginger root, Jerusalem artichokes, Leeks, Mushrooms, Onions, Parsnips, Potatoes, Radishes, Rice, Seaweed of all types, Sweet potatoes, Turnips, Yams

3)Oil (1 to 2 tablespoons on food or by mouth): Ghee, Olive Oil, Garlic oil, Peanut oil

4)Liquids (juices): Beet, Carrot, Pineapple

5)Vitamins and Minerals (derived from the above foods)

BEFORE BED: Mix a drink with whole leaf aloe vera juice and pineapple juice. One ounce of 100 percent agave tequila may be added occasionally for your stomach's sake, not your head's. One hundred percent agave tequila contains vitamin C, which survives the distillation process.

In ZONE THREE, always cook the following foods: Asparagus, Cactus, Eggs, Mushrooms, Peanuts, Potatoes (high in vitamin C after cooking)

CROSSOVER: 11:30 a.m. to 12 noon and 5:30 p.m. to 6 p.m.

CROSSOVER is a half-hour window of time when the transition from one light zone to the next occurs. When you start to change your dietary habits, crossover is an opportunity to eat your favorite food combinations that might not strictly fit Solar guidelines. You can use this time to work with a food you crave until you satisfy the craving or think of an alternative.

For example: If you enjoy an omelet at dinner with toast, eat it at 5:30 p.m. During crossover you can digest the eggs and the grain in the toast.

A FEW BASICS

Stock your pantry with a few basics. These items help make food preparation more simple and healthful.

- Tamari, preferably wheat-free.
- Oils. Buy quality, cold-pressed oils such as olive and sesame. The human brain is only 2 percent of our body weight, yet it consumes 25 percent of the body's oxygen and glucose in the blood. The brain is 60 percent fat. It needs the right kind of oil to feed it. Make sure to include oil with every meal for your brain's well-being.
- Ghee. Most health food stores sell ghee, but if you cannot find it, you can make your own. Buy organic, unsalted butter. Melt the butter in a pan on low heat on the stove top or in the oven. After the butter melts, skim the white layer off the top and discard. Cool the remaining oil and refrigerate until solid. Rinse off the milky residue on the bottom of the solidified butter under the faucet. The remaining product is ghee, or clarified butter.
- Honey. Raw and unfiltered is preferred.
- Apple Cider Vinegar. Be sure it is made from apples and not just *flavored*. Apple cider vinegar is a helpful addition for multiple uses.

• Spices. Keep cayenne, coriander, cumin, ground ginger, garlic powder, turmeric, and the powdered sea vegetables such as nori, dulce, and kelp handy.

• Herbs. If possible, grow a few fresh herbs in your garden or window box. Good herbs to have on hand are garlic chives, onion chives, parsley, sage, oregano, tarragon, and thyme.

• Drink purified water ONE-HALF HOUR *BEFORE* EATING. Do not drink with meals. Wait approximately one to two hours after eating, then drink when you are thirsty. Drinking water in this time frame encourages food assimilation and body hydration. Water flushes out toxins from the system and hydrates the CELLS. Next to air, water is the most important substance in the body. We are mostly water, and we should put the best water possible into our bodies. Drink purified or distilled water. Avoid tap water. Hydrate nuts and dried fruits in distilled water only.

FOOD PREPARATION

Caution: Avoid using aluminum cookware and heating food in aluminum foil. Aluminum can leach into your food and cause heavy metal accumulation.

BROWN RICE:

You can prepare any amount of rice for any number of people when you follow this rule of thumb.

Select a saucepan of appropriate size for the necessary quantity of rice. Pour rice in the pan up to one-third of its depth. Rinse and drain thoroughly. Add distilled water. When the water level goes above the rice, put your thumb on the top of the rice and bring the water level to the first joint in your thumb. Add a small amount of ghee. Place the pot on a burner at high temperature and bring it to a boil. Stir and lower the heat to simmer. Cover and cook approximately 40 minutes or until the water is completely absorbed.

COOKING METHOD:

You can use the following cooking procedure for any kind of vegetable you want to prepare. This method helps preserve flavor and nutrients.

Wash all produce well. Slice the vegetables in half lengthwise, then cut it into one-eighth to one-quarter inch slices on a 45 degree diagonal slant.

In a skillet or large sauce pan, add about one-quarter inch of water to completely cover the bottom of the pan, along with a small amount of oil or ghee.

Bring to a boil. Add your chopped vegetables and cook on high for 10 minutes. Stir occasionally. Do not let the pan boil dry. Add a little water if needed.

When finished cooking, there should be a slight amount of water left in the skillet. Remove from the heat and add seasonings.

SOLAR SEASONINGS:

You season your food immediately after it has cooked and before dextranizing. Of course, you can use any seasonings you like or none at all. For those who want to practice eating Solar in the strictest sense and want to season their food in accord with the food's time zone, here are some suggestions.

Mid-day vegetables:

Broccoli—ghee, oregano, garlic chives

Cauliflower—ghee, salt, coriander

Eggplant—sage, hot sesame oil, tamari

Kale—sesame oil, tamari, cayenne

Summer squash—tamari and thyme

Winter squash—ghee, tamari, hint of cardamom

DEXTRANIZE:

When you finish cooking your food, always dextranize. Dextranizing helps break down the starches into sugars and makes the food easier to digest.

To dextranize, heat the oven to a temperature between 180 and 200 degrees. Place your prepared food in the oven for at least fifteen minutes and up to two hours. Cover the food to hold in moisture.

SUBSTITUTIONS:

Think of new ways to flavor foods in accord with the time zone. Use the tops of green onions for onion flavor in ZONE TWO cooking. Garlic chives give a subtle hint of garlic in noontime dishes.

Look at your recipes and see if you can create a new way to make it fit in the right time frame. Creativity is the way to work with on time eating.

BLESS IT:

Situations arise when you eat out of time. Always pause and acknowledge your act, then bless the food you are about to eat. Blessing food is important when being served by people unaware of Solar eating. Do not insult the person sharing the food they prepare. Thank them, bless it, and enjoy.

Blessing your food (even eaten on time) is always a good practice. Eating Solar is a meditative lifestyle. Nonetheless, please DO NOT ABUSE the privilege of blessing things out of time for convenience sake. If you abuse it, you will block Nature's creative WAY to teach you how to transform your CELLS.

After eating out of time, prepare yourself a drink of apple cider vinegar and honey. This will help relieve any excess intestinal gas. Warm a cup of distilled water, add two teaspoons of apple cider vinegar, and a teaspoon of honey.

Apple cider vinegar is a good all-purpose purifier. Do not drink it in the morning. Only have it in the afternoon and evening. Limit yourself to two cups a day.

For toxic air from gas fumes or second-hand smoke, you can prepare a snuff bottle of apple cider vinegar. Take a small amber-colored bottle and fill it with cotton balls. Soak the cotton balls with apple cider vinegar until the cotton balls are barely wet. Cover. When you are exposed to airborne toxins, open the bottle and sniff deeply. Apple cider vinegar will help clear the pollutants from your lungs.

IT DOESN'T FIT!

Some foods are appropriate for the guidelines of Solar, and others simply do not adapt. What do you do? The lunar cycle is an opportunity to satisfy cravings for favorite non-Solar dishes. Solar eating is a permissive process, a slow, organic change in behavior.

You will stop eating some foods for different reasons. Remember, you are not on a diet, or dieting. You practice a lifestyle.

As some foods drop away, you will find new foods to replace them. Solar is not about denial. Eating Solar is about learning, growing, and changing. Change develops your intellect and increases your immunity. Metamorphic nutrition involves cellular transformation, not dogmatic bullheadedness. It is a process, not a goal or a religion or an -ism. The word *religion* comes from the Latin word *relegare*, which means "to bind up" or "to tie down." Relegare is the Latin root for the English word *regulate*. Looking at these definitions, we can see that religions were formed to control society and individuals. The Solar lifestyle is just the opposite of a religion, for the Solar process is designed to untie your CELLS from the knot of delusions that bind you. Try not to become fixated into a certain set of beliefs or practices. The five Solar rules are tools, guidelines, a place to start. If you are actually living a Solar lifestyle, you will find that you have to be flexible and constantly change. Fixation and dogmatic bullheadedness lead to stagnation, regression, and death. Always be open to change, for that is the nature of life.

BE CREATIVE:

Shopping for foods can sometimes be frustrating. It is more important to find fresh, healthful vegetables, than buy something that fits a recipe, yet has no Vital Life Force. Consider your choices and think about what you can prepare with the best selections available. You might be surprised how wonderfully the foods in the same time zone blend together. Timing takes time to learn, so be patient with yourself. The inspiration will come.

A FEW REMINDERS

Four things to AVOID AT ALL TIMES:

1) Popcorn
2) Melted cheese
3) Deep-fried foods
4) Carbonated beverages

Most chips and crackers are deep-fried. If you want to eat chips or crackers, make sure the package states that they are BAKED.

Soups are a good solution to blend different vegetables and create a complete meal.

A breakfast smoothie is a quick way to start the day. Put your soaked fruits and nuts in a blender, add liquid from the soaking water or use purified water, include the morning oil, cover, and give it a whirl.

Vary your diet. Avoid eating the same food for more than three consecutive days. If you eat too much of the same food, day after day, your body may rebel, and react unfavorably to it. A varied diet gives you a wide variety of vitamins and minerals, the building blocks of health.

Vitamins are now accepted and established as necessary for health and well-being. Biochemists and medical researchers now clearly understand the roles of the different vitamins in the body.

Vitamins seem to offer the "kick" to the minerals that enter our bodies. They work with enzymes, or as parts of enzymes, to create and control the energy and protein by-products of cells. They work with minerals and hydrocarbon molecules building and maintaining a perfect body. (Jensen, p.280)

EXCEPTIONAL FOODS

The following foods are neutral. Eat them as shown.

Noon or night	Anytime
apple cider vinegar	brown rice
tamari and miso (traditional)	clarified butter (ghee)
tofu	honey
	olive oil

BLOOD TYPE

Your BODY is the church HEALTH lives in. In agricultural times, spiritual teachers referred to the BODY as a temple with nine visible doors and one invisible door. The nine visible doors are; two eyes, two ears, two nostrils, your mouth, your anus, and your sex opening. The invisible door is your pituitary gland, the master gland, whose prime function is to stabilize your metabolism.

When we were born, oxygen came in our nose and hit the pituitary gland, which set the timing for our body. Life doesn't interact with an individual until the breath goes through the nostrils. Scientists have discovered that three and one-half ounces of oxygen in our lungs produce the phenomenon called consciousness.

After we breathe, we start to eat. We take in vitamins and minerals. As explained in the fourth rule of Solar, all minerals are electromagnetic except iron and carbon. Iron and carbon are magnetic only. Nature runs our body on magnetic energy in the form of iron stored in the pituitary gland. Iron is a prime element in the body and is the only mineral able to regulate metabolism. Iron is extracted from magnetite found in the pituitary gland. Iron attracts oxygen. Oxygen cleans and filters the blood through the heart, lungs, and liver.

After iron and carbon, we have the electromagnetic minerals; 108 functional minerals and 36 radical minerals. In agricultural times, the radical minerals were pictured as devils and gargoyles on church structures. (Remember, for the ancients, the church represented the human body.) Radicals attack basic minerals. If trace minerals do not go in on time, the body is vulnerable to radical invasion. To stay healthy, you must eat foods with trace minerals and basic minerals on time. Basic and trace minerals operate under the same rules: TIME is the important factor.

Elements taken in the same light zone electromagnetically interrelate to each other, which allows the body to constrict and dilate on time. All concerns about the metabolism of vitamins and minerals can be worked out by proper food combination in the correct time frame. Pills are not the answer. Artificial vitamins are often made from abnormal and inorganic substances. Also, pills have vitamins and/or minerals from different light zones in indigestible combinations not found in nature at dosages many times the needed amount. Hence, they do not metabolize and may create more health problems.

To improve metabolism, it helps to know your blood type. If you eat inappropriately for your blood type at the right time, you may experience acidosis or alkalosis. If you eat suitable foods for your blood type at the right time, you will accelerate the cleaning up process with less discomfort. The object of eating on time is to clean up our acts, so we should work with our blood type as much as possible.

If you are a positive (+) blood type, you are considered "hyper". If you are a negative (-) blood type, you are considered "hypo". Hyper types will absorb their food faster and hypo types will absorb their food slower. If you are a hyper type and find yourself going too fast, Adano gave us a simple technique to slow ourselves down. You can put your right fist under your left armpit, squeeze, and breathe out. Conversely, if you are a hypo type and find yourself going too slow and want to speed up, you can put your left fist under your right armpit, squeeze, and breathe out.

Plus (+) and minus (-) types A and AB can eat a 100 percent fiber diet and suffer no ill effects. A 100 percent fiber diet is pure vegetarian. Often, types A and AB will develop acidosis if they eat meat habitually. You can tell if you have acidosis by looking at your tongue. An acidosis tongue is heavily coated. To balance an acidic condition, eat more raw and unrefined foods.

Plus (+) and minus (-) types B and O can eat a 100 percent tissue (meat) diet and suffer no ill effects. If a type O eats a 100 percent fiber (vegetarian) diet, they are prone to develop alkalosis. An alkalosis tongue is pink and dry. To balance an over alkaline condition, eat more cooked and refined foods.

Awareness of your blood type allows you to make appropriate choices about fiber and tissue foods. Know your blood type, integrate this information with eating on time, and you will achieve the maximum benefit.

BUYER BE AWARE

Transnational agrochemical companies have opened Pandora's box by developing, planting, and releasing genetically engineered foods called GMOs (genetically modified organisms) and GEOs (genetically engineered organisms). GMOs threaten human development, are contrary to Nature, and are a direct attack on Solar eating. How can you eat on time when you eat the DNA of a tomato spliced with bacteria, viruses, and flounder genes? The Environmental Protection Agency (EPA) classifies some genetically engineered corn and potatoes as pesticides rather than vegetables!

The carbon-based body is not designed to eat manmade genetic abominations that make us stupid. "The crops are actually less nutritious—they lacked essential trace elements and minerals, particularly iron and zinc. A reduction in IQ of 10 points was also observed in the generation of children who were brought up on these [GE] foods." (Ticciati and Ticciati, p.46)

Humans and the Earth are one and the same. In 1851 Chief Seattle of the Suquamish and other Native American tribes around Washington's Puget Sound delivered one of the most profound environmental statements ever made. His powerful words still remind us:

> . . . We are part of the earth and it is part of us . . . Whatever befalls the earth befalls the sons of the earth . . . This we know: The earth does not belong to man; man belongs

to the earth. All things are connected. We may be brothers after all. We shall see. One thing we know which the white man may one day discover: Our God is the same God.

You may think now that you own Him as you wish to own our land; but you cannot. He is the God of man, and His compassion is equal for the red man and the white. This earth is precious to Him, and to harm the earth is to heap contempt on its Creator. The whites too shall pass; perhaps sooner than all other tribes. Contaminate your bed and you will one night suffocate in your own waste.

The environment and humankind have developed together for millions of years. Right when humanity stands on the edge of a quantum leap in conscious awareness, geneticists attack the DNA, the hard drive containing the Diamond Body Program. Break the hard drive and the programs are lost. If scientists change Nature's genetics, they change human genetics. As already mentioned, we are thrown into the environment to learn how to synchronize with It, not the other way around. A WAY to synchronize with the environment is to eat on time. If geneticists alter our food's genes, the environment our DNA lives in will not trigger the gene in the same way, thus jeopardizing humanity's chance to develop conscious awareness.

Genetic engineers cut genes (segments of DNA) out of plants, animals, viruses, and bacteria and insert them into unrelated plants and animals, fundamentally altering Nature's creation. These genetic experiments result in manmade organisms never before seen on Earth. Once these "frankenfoods" are released into the environment, they can never be recalled.

When the genetic engineer moves genes from one organism to another, the gene is inserted into the DNA of the target organism at random. As a consequence, there is a risk the inserted gene may disrupt the functioning of other genes in the target organism essential to the life of that organism. Yet the agrochemical transnational companies cover over the risks with slogans and simplifications. At best, this technology is imprecise, at worst it is criminal. GEOs are unpredictable. No one knows what the long term consequences might be. Furthermore, GMO foods offer no advantage. Our food is fine just the way Nature created it. In fact, Nature's food is perfect. To change perfection invites disaster.

The dangers of GMO foods are a matter of living to live or living to die. For example: "In 1989, a genetically engineered form of the food supplement tryptophan contained toxic contaminants. As a result, 37 people died, 1,500 were permanently disabled, and 5,000 others became very ill." (Ticciati and Ticciati, p.7) Tryptophan in its natural form is perfectly safe. The genetically engineered tryptophan killed people.

In 1996, there were 13 GE products approved for commercial distribution. In 2002, there were over 40 GE products on the market including corn, flax, squash, soybeans, canola, papaya, potatoes, radicchio, tomatoes, sugar beets, and cotton oils. Over 70 percent of the processed foods in the United States contain genetically engineered ingredients such as corn, soy, canola, and cotton oils. "U. S. food companies use gene-altered corn and soybeans in more than two-thirds of their processed foods." (Hart, p.19) The amount of foods with genetically altered ingredients is increasing so fast, it will not be long before all our foods are corrupted.

A toxicologist who worked in one of the government's regulatory agencies for 13 years said:

> This technology [genetic engineering] is being promoted, in the face of concerns by respectable scientists and in the face of data to the contrary, by the very agencies which are supposed to be protecting human health and the environment. The bottom line, in my view, is that we are confronted with the most powerful technology the world has ever known, and it is being rapidly deployed with almost no thought what-so-ever to its consequences. (qtd. in Ticciati and Ticciati, p.14)

Dairy products from cows injected with a genetically altered hormone called recombinant bovine growth hormone (rBGH developed by Monsanto) and animals fed with genetically engineered grain that is unfit for human consumption (StarLink corn developed by AgrEvo) are on the market without any labeling. Recombinant bovine growth hormone in milk raises the levels of IGF-1 hormone in humans who drink it and can "increase people's chances of contracting breast cancer and colon cancer." (Hart, p.42) In May

1998, the "prestigious scientific publication, the British journal *Lancet*, reported that premenopausal women with higher blood levels of IGF-1 are seven times more likely to develop breast cancer than are women with lower levels of IGF-1." (Hart, p.43)

Britain, together with Japan and the entire European Union, have banned the import and sale of GMO food products in their countries. Yet most Americans remain ignorant of the obvious dangers inherent in GMOs, because the dangers of GMO foods are blacked-out from the American media. If the occasional story makes it to the media, it is decidedly favorable agrochemical propaganda. Corporate buyouts and consolidation of media outlets in the 1990's resulted in more coverage of sex scandals, entertainment news, and terrorist scare mongering than reporting on public policy issues such as the food we eat, the water we drink, and the air we breathe.

For example, in 1998, America was in a frenzy about President Clinton's sexual escapades with White House intern Monica Lewinsky. As the media distracted Americans with such silliness, the transnational agrochemical companies quietly planted millions of acres of gene-altered crops on American soil. Since the destruction of the twin towers in New York City on September 11, 2001, nightly television news programs traumatize Americans with daily threats of terror. Yet behind the scenes, obscured from public view, the Bush administration is in the process of approving the first genetically engineered fish. If approved, these fish will be allowed to swim in the open waters and be sold in supermarkets without any mandatory labeling. The Center for Food Safety writes:

> Studies by scientists at Purdue University show that GE fish, due to their larger size, have a mating advantage over native fish. Unfortunately, the offspring of GE fish have a one-third greater mortality rate because of the impacts of the added genetic material. With these findings the Purdue scientists predict that the introduction of GE fish would cause extinction of native species within only a few generations. (www.centerforfoodsafety.org)

How can you protect yourself? First and most importantly, insist that the food you buy is labeled with GE ingredients clearly identified. Contact your political representatives and local grocers. Push for mandatory labels on genetically engineered foods. You have a right to know what you are eating. Next, search out foods that are organically produced. By purchasing organic foods, you are supporting local, sustainable farmers. Support food companies that avoid GE foods.

Read the labels on the food you buy. Greenpeace offers a "True Food" shopping list online at www.truefoodnow.org or you can call 1-800-219-9260 and they will mail you one. The Greenpeace True Food Shopping List tells you what is genetically engineered and what isn't. Mothers for Natural Law offer a good food list on their website, www.safe-food.org. You can call Mothers for Natural Law at 1-614-472-2499, or write them at P.O. Box 1177, Fairfield, Iowa,

52556. Keep in mind, if the label mentions corn, canola, soybeans, cottonseed oil, potatoes, tomatoes, dairy products, animal products, or papaya without explicitly qualifying it as non-GMO, then the product probably contains genetically engineered ingredients. Even with a food list, you have no way of knowing for sure if the food contains GMOs unless the food itself is labeled.

Consumers should be allowed to choose what they put into their mouths. Take charge of your food. Know what you are eating and when to eat it. Demand that foods with GE ingredients are labeled accordingly.

MAHASANA

Guru means teacher in Sanskrit. In agricultural times, a student or disciple sought out a guru for instruction on how to free one's self from life's illusion. They called it freedom, *moksha,* enlightenment, or liberation. A spiritual teacher would initiate the student and show them which line to get in. The teacher gave the initiate spiritual practices to do while they waited. If the initiate faithfully did their practices, they kept their place in line. The line slowly progressed, just as any line does to anything. Gradually, perhaps over many lifetimes, the student learned that if they waited long enough, their turn to face the reality of their CELLS would come.

Even though waiting is the highest science, most students lose patience and look for a faster way. So the student finds another guru who promises quicker results. Having initiations with different spiritual Masters is like changing checkout lines in the supermarket. When you switch lines, you lose your place and start over. The new checkout line may be faster or slower than the previous one. Still, you must wait your turn and deal with your own unique challenges until you are ready to face your CELLS, or **What** you are.

Whether you follow a guru or not, all change happens in your body. The spiritual life, indeed all existence involves physical, cellular, biological change. Bodily change is a scientifically validated fact, not a philosophical idea. Because God is pure HEALTH, our body is our best guru. Creative intelligence gave us a carbon-based body to work with and learn from, here and now, on planet Earth. Furthermore, we can only live NOW, and NOW is the most fantastic *present* for two reasons.

1)Our body is a birthday present from creative Intelligence and the greatest gift in the universe. Of all the body types in creation, our carbon-based body is uniquely set up to become something entirely new.

2)We breathe and live here and now, in the present moment. If we let the present slip by and do nothing to improve ourselves, we will miss an opportunity. And when life passes us by, we will have to find another body to live in. We never know what we will get in the next life, so it benefits us to work with our CELLS now while we are still breathing.

Most people, like the caterpillar who eats itself to death, wait too long before they realize they let the greatest gift in the universe, the present, slip away.

Your body is smarter than your intellect. If you listen to your body, it will guide you to the highest fulfillment in life; the diamond body. If you listen to your intellect it will be like "the blind leading the blind" (Matthew 15:14) and you will fall into the ditch of ignorance; ignoring **What** you are.

When you start listening to your body and following your path into the deepest recesses of your CELLS, you face the reality of living in the NOW. Eating your meditation places you in the present, by being aware of every bite of food you put into your mouth and every word you speak out of it.

Solar eaters work with renunciation—not by renouncing the ways of the world to live in a cave in the forest—but by renouncing foods that harm their body and eating foods that support health. Eating Solar is a cosmic reality and a science of living that helps to build our bodies into the immortal diamond body. The Bible metaphorically defines the diamond body as "a building of God, a house not made with hands, eternal in the heavens." (2 Corinthians 5:1) The Rig Veda viii, 19 states, "Let this mortal clay [body] be the immortal God."

These statements meant something to ancient agricultural societies. Agricultural thinking motivated the masses to improve themselves through guilt. Today we live in a mechanical society and use technical language to express our ideas. Therefore, our thinking demands a more rational approach than guilt to motivate us to change. The antiquated science of the Bible and Judeo-Christian guilt no longer inspires us to improve ourselves.

Technical language does not produce guilt, it provides the opportunity for commitment. Technical language forces you to commit yourself to act what you say like in the Old West where your word is your bond. When it comes to working with cosmic Law, our word is all we have to bargain with. Technical language demands we do what we say. LIFE asks us to confront and realize our CELLS by commitment and action, rather than guilt.

To that end, Adano gave us one yoga posture. He stood facing us with his arms at his sides, palms facing forward, legs spread apart, and his feet firmly planted on the ground. He said, "This is *Mahasana*. It means, stand on your own two feet."

Adano refused to be our guru. Instead, he encouraged us to let go of guru worship, something for nothing consciousness, and seeking God outside ourselves. To seek for God is to avoid It. Searching for God outside your CELLS is akin to looking for your glasses when they sit on the end of your nose! Seeking for something you already have is futile, like a dog chasing its own tail. Furthermore, no one, not even a guru, can give you what you already have.

Adano urged us to stand on our own two feet (Mahasana), cleanup our CELLS (eat Solar and cleanup with hydropathy), be our own guru and disciple (know what and when we eat), and speak the utmost to our CELLS (use the power of sonics to transform our lives). In this way, we learn to work with the environment rather than fighting against It. We allow synchronicity (God) to work for us.

Creative intelligence asks us to deal with the pressure and frustrations in life to reconcile our personality (the **who**) with our divine nature (the **What**). As long as we live and breathe in a carbon-based body, creative Intelligence gives us every opportunity to unlock the Diamond Body Program in our DNA.

ADANO and SOLAR NUTRITION

Question: "What do you do for a living?"
Adano: "I eat on time."

Adano C. Ley was born on December 9, 1924, near Georgetown, British Guyana (now named Guyana) in South America. In his youth, Adano trained to become a Catholic priest. Soon into his training, he began to question the catechism. The church claimed he was too much of a mystic and declared him unfit for the priesthood, so he left.

At 15, Adano received his inheritance. A few years later, he moved to Montreal, Canada, where he eventually bought two restaurants and became a successful restaurateur.

In his spare time, Adano ran the Montreal Self-Realization Fellowship center, founded by Paramahansa Yogananda, who deeply influenced Adano's spiritual thinking. Adano wanted to find God fast, so he asked for all his karma.

On June 22, 1955, Adano went to a friend's house to help him install a television antenna. While on the roof, Adano slipped and fell to the ground. He died, yet remained conscious. He experienced the different vibrational after-death states and pushed through them until he realized **What** he was.

Adano explained, "All your karma is total cash on the line. Cash it in, right here and now. I learned that the easiest way to find God is to die. If He allows you to breathe again, you're lucky. That's the way I had to learn, because I'm hardheaded. They used to call me nitty-gritty. I can't believe it until I prove it, and then I prove it and still don't believe it. So that's the problem with me."

In the subspace realm, he saw Saints and Masters watching him. The wonderful beings who watched gave him one instruction. They said telepathically with their eyes, 'BREATHE!' But he could not breathe sitting in the subspace realm. He had to get back into his physical body to breathe.

Adano faced an agonizing decision. He could have a "cosmic vacation" (as he called it) and stay in the subspace realm. If he did, he would have to go through another birth. If he chose rebirth, he would lose his memory and he wanted to keep it. To keep his memory, he had to return to his broken body lying on the street. Obviously, he did not want to do that.

As he struggled with his predicament, cosmic Intelligence showed him a vision. He saw himself as a kite flying in a clear blue sky. Attached to the kite was a long tail waving in the breeze.

Strangely, the tail of the kite contained the faces of those currently living on Earth who needed his help. Cosmic Intelligence offered him a way out. It said, "Once you finish helping the last person on the tail of the kite, your work on Earth is finished. You can come back to ME."

Adano carefully looked at each face on the kite's tail and agreed to serve.

He asked for all his karma and he had to live it. He had to accept his broken and bleeding body lying on the street, which was numb from the impact. The numbness was quickly traveling to his head and he knew if it reached his head, it would be over. So he put his hand in his mouth and bit as hard as he could, but he felt nothing. Finally, the first sensation of pain came in his hand. He continued biting, and the numbness gradually retreated to his toes. Pain brought his spirit back into his physical body. The pain also kept him alive until the ambulance arrived.

Adano died again during the ambulance ride to the hospital. He said later, "People die because they panic. I pushed through the death experience without panic. And I'll tell you this much, if you're in an ambulance and your body is all broken up, that siren is no asset. It'll panic you quicker than anything. They blow the siren to help people get out of the way, letting them go faster. They think the siren will get you there on time. But, it'll kill you before you get there, because your body panics and shuts down!"

When Adano arrived at the hospital, the doctors and nurses revived him. The fall broke most of the bones in his body, his lungs were full of fluid, and his breaths were shallow. They rushed him into surgery. Adano died a third time on the operating table, yet lived to tell about it. He said, "I saw the comedy of this whole phenomenon called LIFE. I laughed to myself, and gave control of my body to the doctors. I said to myself, 'Oh come on man, this is so well-planned out by Creative Intelligence, you don't have a single thing to do with the survival of your mechanism other than live it.' To one who becomes aware of it, you see the whole plan right in front of you. You have to let go and let God take charge. You must allow this Principle to work, while you observe."

After surgery, he found himself bound in a full-body cast. He laid in his hospital bed "like a chicken on a spit" for over a year. Still, his bones refused to knit. Adano realized that if he was ever going to leave the hospital, he would have to heal himself. All he could do was eat, so he experimented with food as a therapy to heal his broken bones. He began with an egg. He asked for an egg for breakfast, an egg for lunch, and an egg for dinner. The nurses thought he was crazy, but Adano was determined. He noticed that the egg gave him gas at breakfast and lunch, yet digested fine at dinner. He experimented with other foods, one at a time, and recorded the results. He discovered that when he ate was just as important as what he ate. Over the next year, through trial and error, he healed himself eating foods on time.

Adano needed to metabolize minerals to repair his broken bones. On time eating gave his body the minerals it needed in the right time frame for complete absorption. Adano coined the term Solar Nutrition for eating on time. He recognized that we are manifestations of light and sound playing the charade of eating and sleeping. He understood that we ingest light when we eat, and it is the light that sustains us, not the food. Unknown to him, he had stumbled on an ancient initiatic science.

After spending two years in a full body cast, he was finally free to walk into life again. Adano opened a clinic in Houston, Texas, where he served Solar meals, gave specialized colonics, offered reflexology treatments, gave instructions in transformational techniques, and held group meditation in the evenings.

In 1969, Adano attended a lecture given by Swami Ananda Saraswati of New Delhi, India. He was one of Mahatma Gandhi's aids during India's struggle for independence. Swami Ananda Saraswati knew **What** he was. When Swami Ananda saw Adano walk into the room, he abruptly stopped his lecture and said to a startled Adano, "I'm going to make you a Swami right now!"

Swami Ananda immediately performed an initiation ceremony to make Adano a Swami and give him his spiritual name. He considered naming Adano, Swami Adyananda, meaning "One Eternal Now Bliss" or "First Spirit", until he realized that only God could have such a title. So he named Adano, Swami Nityananda Saraswati, meaning "Ever New Bliss." Adano preferred to call himself "Swami

Nitty-Gritty", because he focused on the nitty-gritty issues of food and elimination.

Over the years, Adano continued to improve his novel transformational techniques. He traveled around the country teaching Solar classes, cooking Solar meals, selling Solar products, and sharing his most recent discoveries. The powerful combination of eating Solar and colon hydropathy was the backbone of Adano's cellular regeneration program. He wanted to have his unique colon lavage device installed in clinics across the country, but it was not to be.

On October 11, 1989, Adano finished teaching a Solar class in Virginia and was scheduled to return to Houston. Yet, he knew he had helped the last person from the tail of the kite. With his duties on Earth done, he quietly walked upstairs, went into the bathroom, sat on the toilet, and left his physical carbon-based body to live in his subspace diamond body.

The clinic in Houston closed shortly after.

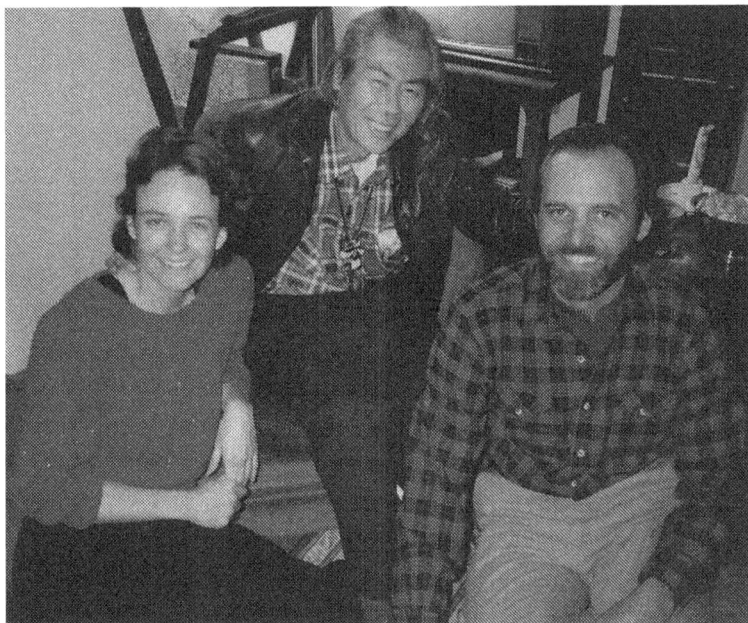

Linda, Adano, and Steven
Santa Fe, New Mexico, December 1988

LIST OF REFERENCES

Duggan, R.N., Sandra. *Edgar Cayce's Guide to Colon Care*. Virginia Beach: Inner Vision, 1995

Gray, Robert. *The Colon Health Handbook* (12th Rev. ed.). Reno, NV: Emerald Publishing, 1991.

Hart, Kathleen. *Eating in the Dark*. New York: Pantheon Books, 2002.

Jensen, D.C., Bernard. *Nature Has A Remedy*. Lincolnwood, Ill: Keats Publishing, 2001

Kime, M.D., Zane R. *Sunlight*. Penryn, CA: World Health Publications, 1980.

Schlosser, Eric. *Fast Food Nation*. New York: Houghton Mifflin Company, 2001.

Ticciati, Laura and Robin Ticciati, Ph.D. *Genetically Engineered Foods— Are they safe? You decide*. Chicago: NTC/Contemporary Publishing, 1998.

Tilden, M.D., J. H. *Toxemia Explained*. Mokelumne Hill, CA: Health Research, 1960.

NOTES

NOTES

NOTES

www.ingramcontent.com/pod-product-compliance
Lightning Source LLC
Chambersburg PA
CBHW031212270326
41931CB00006B/527